# Believe It or Not!
# TRUE
# Emergency Room Stories

## by Kevin Pezzi, M.D.

### Editor: Karla Lewk

*a Transcope Publication*

# Believe It or Not!
# TRUE
# Emergency Room Stories

# *Acknowledgments*

I am indebted to my editor, Karla Lewk, for her tireless devotion to the polishing of this book. I am also grateful to my colleagues for their contributions. And last, but certainly not least, I wish to thank you, the reader, for choosing this book.

## Other books by Dr. Pezzi:

*Fascinating Health Secrets*
*Fascinating Weight Loss & Beauty Secrets*
*Fascinating Sex Secrets*
*The Cellulite & Wrinkle Eraser*

## Visit the Transcope web site at http://www.transcope.com

In it you will find:

Excerpts from Dr. Pezzi's *Fascinating Health Secrets*

Other Transcope products

A link to Dr. Pezzi's personal web page (*there's nothing else like it!*)

### *Do you have an interesting ER story?*

If your submission is accepted for publication, you will receive *free* the next edition of the book and tape which bears your story *or*, if you prefer, a current copy of the book and tape. Please specify your choice. Along with your submission, please state that this material is unpublished, and that you are authorizing its publication by Transcope, Inc., which will then own the copyright to the material in exchange for the compensation given above. Stories may be edited for length, clarity, spelling, punctuation, and so forth. If you include any names, change them so that even I don't know the identity of the patient. Send your submission(s) to kpezzi@transcope.com or mail them to Transcope, Inc., 955 Nature Trail, Holly, MI 48442. *Thank you!*

---

# *About the Author*

After graduating in the top 1% of his class from Wayne State University School of Medicine, Dr. Pezzi practiced emergency medicine for 11 years.

He enjoys snowmobiling, riding his Sea-doo®, inventing, thinking, shopping, baking, dating, bicycling, exercising, watching movies, traveling, working in his shop, shooting, being outdoors, reading, and of course writing.

# *Introduction*

"Is this the emergency room, or the *Twilight Zone*?" The latter two words were emphasized as if that were the only viable option.

I had been writing orders at the nurses' station, and looked up to find Mr. Singer shaking his head in disbelief. He had been in the ER for several hours as he waited for his wife to be admitted to the hospital's cardiac care unit. This provided him with the opportunity to witness a variety of bizarre events.

"I don't know," I responded, "I often wonder the same thing myself."

"Before today, I thought all you guys did was treat emergencies."

"I wish . . ." I ruefully replied.

"Never would I have guessed that things like this go on in an ER," he said.

"That's what I tell myself every day, Mr. Singer. Just when I think I've seen it all, I'll have a patient who proves me wrong."

---

In this book, you will meet scores of patients who left me—a seasoned ER doctor—saying to myself, "I can't believe it!" After reading this book, I'm sure you will be saying the same thing to yourself.

These stories focus upon the unusual aspects of each particular case, and rarely delve into the specifics of medical or surgical treatment. The intriguing nature of these cases lies not in catheter sizes and other bits of medical minutiae, but rather in the unique interplay between the ER staff, the patient, and heaven knows who or what else.

Curiously, books of this genre which concentrate upon emergencies fail to accurately convey the spirit and pulse of real emergency rooms. That's because ER patients often have no problem which can be construed to be an emergency. While they may have no pressing medical problems, they often present with interesting cases. In fact, there is often an inverse correlation between the seriousness of a case and its uniqueness. In my opinion, it is that latter element which provides the fodder for some highly captivating stories.

One of my goals in writing this book was to give you an idea of what it is like to be a real ER doctor in a real ER. To achieve this end, I have sometimes appended my opinions to the stories. As you will see, my views have been influenced by repeated exposure to events which are outrageous, maddening, and just plain wacky. But that's the reality of a real ER; to ignore it is to miss an integral aspect of its quintessence.

This book is a window into another world—the world of emergency medicine. Entering this strange world will undoubtedly leave an indelible impression upon you, as it has me.

Enjoy.


Kevin Pezzi, M.D.
Somewhere in northern Michigan
April 3, 1998

# *Contents*

# Believe It or Not! TRUE Emergency Room Stories

It has been said that truth is stranger than fiction. The following stories, all of which are true, lend credence to that belief.

## *Surprise!*

■ The nurse seemed anxious. Handing me the chart, she said, "You'd better see this patient right away, Dr. Pezzi." I thought about asking her why, but I assumed I'd find out soon enough.

"*Hiiiiiii*, I'm Eric!" he exclaimed as he extended his blood-soaked hand to greet me. I declined to shake his bloody hand, but this didn't seem to faze him. He continued, "I'm sure you've seen me before. I was on the cover of *Cosmo* last month!"

Actually, no, I hadn't seen him. And I didn't know that *Cosmopolitan* was in the habit of featuring obese men on their covers. Every *Cosmo* I'd ever seen had a slim, drop-dead gorgeous woman as the cover model. He didn't fit the description.

The patient came to the ER for repair of a finger cut, which I examined. "I'll need to suture it," I explained.

"Oh, no, that will take too long! Can't you just glue it?" he responded.

At that time, no surgical glues were in use in the United States. "Glue it? With what?" I asked.

"Oh, whatever you've got . . . Elmer's®, a glue stick, I don't care."

"I'm sorry, we don't glue cuts together. This will need suturing."

He seemed genuinely disappointed. "But I'm in a hurry! Suturing will take too long!"

I asked why he was in a hurry. "I'm flying on the Concorde. I'm meeting Jackie O. for lunch in Europe." This I gauged to be a tad less than plausible. Also, by considering the time differential between the U.S. and Europe, he'd probably arrive at 3 a.m. I doubted that Mrs. Onassis would be in the mood for lunch at that time.

"I have to take care of this cut," I said.

He seemed to accept this with equanimity. As I was working on the cut, he changed the subject. "Michael Jackson wants me dead," he matter-of-factly revealed.

"What?" I wasn't sure if I'd heard him correctly.

"Yes, it's true. He wants to kill me."

"Why would he want to kill you?"

"Oh, I don't know, but he's said it many times. By the way, do you want my autograph?"

As I placed the bandage on his cut, I said, "Sure. Let me get some paper. I'll be right back."

I decided to commit him. His delusions were fairly innocuous, with the exception of the Michael Jackson fantasy. People who feel threatened sometimes attack the source of the perceived threat, and I was concerned that he might try to strike first. This incident occurred shortly after the attempted assassination of President Reagan by John Hinckley. Hinckley had been seeing a psychiatrist beforehand, and I'd heard that the psychiatrist had some prior knowledge of the assassination ideas which were brewing in Hinckley's mind. The psychiatrist was criticized for failing to take action which may have averted the attack on Reagan. Not wanting to be the subject of similar criticism, I called a psychiatrist. But not Jackie O. I thought she'd understand.

▪ While performing a procedure, I'll often engage in "small talk" with patients. This can dispel some of their apprehension by taking their mind off the procedure, and it makes my job more interesting. The conversation usually follows a predictable pattern, but there are times when I have been floored by their responses. For example, last December I asked a 24-year-old patient if she were going to spend Christmas with her parents. "No," she replied.

I asked, "Why not?"

With little emotion, she said, "My Mom is in jail."

I then asked, "Well, what about your Dad?"

She said, "He's dead."

Pausing a few seconds to collect myself, my curiosity got the best of me. I asked, "Why is your Mom in prison?"

She answered impassively, "She killed my Dad."

■ A middle-aged man, despondent over the breakup with his lover, attempted suicide by swallowing a Bic® pen. He was taken to the ER and rushed into surgery. The surgeon removed the pen, and then used it, writing on the patient's chart, "Writes first time, every time."

■ The patient was explaining how he had received multiple cuts on his body. "First, I installed Lotus' Word Pro on my computer. Then, I kept getting a bunch of GPFs[1] (General Protection Faults), so I reconfigured my *config.sys* and *autoexec.bat* files, then I ran *memmaker*, but none of this seemed to help. The keyboard and mouse would sometimes lockup, so I'd have to do a cold reboot. I spent hours on the phone speaking with Lotus' technical support staff, but they offered little help. To top it off, they wanted to charge me for the privilege of receiving incompetent advice on fixing faults in their buggy program."

With me nodding in sympathy (being a fellow user of Word Pro), he continued. "Every time the computer would crash, I'd lose all of the information that I'd entered since the last time I had saved the file. I would have saved my work more often, but it would take about three minutes for the computer to write the file to the hard drive. So, I was darned if I do, and darned if I don't. I was just trying to get my work done, you know? And every time I turned around, the program was *μ¢#&@! up again! I hired my own computer consultant, but he wasn't able to make much headway—it just cost me more money. I bought some books on computers, and tried to figure it out myself, but nothing I did was of any

---

[1]    GPFs, config.sys, autoexec.bat, memmaker, cold reboot: if you're not into computers (lucky you!), you won't know what these terms mean. However, they're not germane to the understanding of this story. Suffice it to say that they are the vestiges of an arcane, antiquated computer operating system that has caused untold hours of frustration and wasted productivity. Society has showered the Grand Pooh-Bah of this anachronistic execration, Bill Gates of Microsoft, not with condemnation and lawsuits, but with about 51 *billion* dollars, making him the richest man in the world. Go figure.

Mr. Gates claims to be working on this usability problem, but—for all his reputed intelligence and the collective resources of Microsoft—progress is pathetically slow in coming. In my opinion, this is because their tack is incredibly misguided. They believe that computers can be made more user-friendly by making them more complex. For example, they are developing computers with built-in cameras which constantly monitor your facial expressions. If this idiotic idea is ever implemented, it will create more problems than it solves. What Gates needs is not more techno-geeks whose brains are addled with a lust for technology per se, but technologically savvy people who can devise logical, workable ways to enhance usability *now*—not thirty years in the future. Ah, but in the insular world of Microsoft, Gates has shielded himself from this reality by hiring a veritable army of well-paid yes-men, who blindly accede to his dictates, oblivious to their repercussions. Perhaps nothing epitomizes this monkey-see, monkey-do attitude more than the fact that some Microsoft employees have actually adopted a classic Gatesian mannerism: namely, nervously rocking in a chair. If his sycophantic troops willingly adopt his personal mannerisms, it is not surprising that they'll kowtow to his decrees. 51 billion dollars can certainly buy a lot of deference.

help. I wanted to transfer my data to another program, but the export filter wasn't very good, and I would have lost months of work."

While I could easily relate to his frustration, the ER was getting busy, so I was in a hurry to learn how he had received the cuts. Prodding him to get to the crux of the matter, he said, "Look, Doc, I'm a patient man, but enough is enough, right? I've wasted hundreds of hours on that stupid program, and I'm not making much progress. So, tonight, it screws up again, and I've had it. Rather than continue to fritter away my time, I thought it was best to cut my losses, and quit. I did what I've been wanting to do for a long time."

"What's that?" I inquired. Looking around to make sure no one was listening, he confided, "Well, I got out my shotgun, and blasted the damn computer. Gave it both barrels, too. The monitor blew up, and its glass went flying. You're not going to turn me in to the police, are you?"

Nope.

■ A lady in her mid-twenties came to the ER by ambulance, accompanied by her husband. Expecting that she had come in for chest pain, difficulty breathing, or some other potentially serious reason, I immediately went to see her. The conversation didn't exactly conform to what I had in mind.

**Dr. Pezzi:** Hi, I'm Dr. Pezzi. How may I help you?

**Patient:** (smiling) I think my vagina is too loose.

**Dr. Pezzi:** You think your *vagina* is too loose?

**Patient:** Well, I'm not sure. My boyfriend can't satisfy me—you know, he can't make me come—and I don't know if it is because my vagina is too loose, or because he's on crack. He's a drug dealer, and he uses the stuff himself, you know.

**Dr. Pezzi:** (looking at the man sitting mute in the corner) Is this your boyfriend?

**Patient:** No, that's my husband. I don't have sex with my husband, just my boyfriend.

**Dr. Pezzi:** (wondering *What on Earth?*) Do you use any drugs?

**Patient:** No, and I can make myself come when I play with myself. So is it my vagina, or is it that he's on crack? Will you check me and see if it is tight enough?

**Dr. Pezzi:** Your boyfriend's use of crack may indeed contribute to your problem.

**Patient:** You gonna check me now?

**Dr. Pezzi:** No, I'm not. If you had not called for an ambulance, I would have examined you, simply as a courtesy, even though your problem is clearly not an emergency. We have a limited number of ambulances in the county, and an elderly person could be dying from a heart attack at home right now because the ambulance which would have brought them to the hospital was busy transporting you here. Besides, even if I determined that your vagina was loose, it's not as if I would operate on it in the ER.

**Patient:** You wouldn't? *Darn*, I was hoping I could get it fixed today.

**Dr. Pezzi:** That's not what we are here for. You'll need to see a gynecologist.

**Patient:** But I don't want to.

**Dr. Pezzi:** Why not?

**Patient:** 'Cause I'll have to pay him, that's why!

**Husband:** Hey, I'm not payin' for it, either! If I'm not getting it, I sure ain't gonna pay to have it fixed! Your boyfriend can pay the bill!

As Ozzie and Harriet continued their discussion, I excused myself and went to see other patients.

■ Whenever the subject of emergency room stories is discussed, one of the first things that people with ER experience discuss is the subject of rectal foreign bodies. I've never had much affinity for this topic, but I've seen a fair number of patients with such a problem. These stories share a number of similarities, so one story on this subject should suffice.

Bart, age 28, seemed embarrassed as he described the events which caused him to seek emergency treatment. "Well, I was at home . . . uh, naked, you know . . . and I sat on a chair. A light bulb was on the chair—*but I have no idea how it got there!*—and when I sat down, it went inside my butt. It's still there. I couldn't get it out."

Sure enough, the light bulb (a 60-watt GE, in case you're curious) was still inside his rectum. Unfortunately, the bulb had shattered, which was causing Bart to bleed profusely. We stabilized him in the ER, and he was taken to surgery for removal of the glass and repair of the rectal cuts.

Here are the similarities, and the one variable:

**Gender:** I suppose there are a few women out there with—oh, how should I phrase this?—rectal proclivities, but men far outnumber the women.

**Age:** Typically in the horny years, when libido often exceeds brainpower.

**Embarrassment:** It's genuine.

**Wacky story:** Concocted in a futile attempt to deceive the ER doctor into believing that they're a regular Joe. Spare me the embellishment, please. I'm here to treat you, not judge you (scam artists, welfare frauds, and narcotic-seeking junkies excepted).

**Fruitless attempt at removal of said foreign body:** Hoping to circumvent the ER experience, people often resort to drastic measures of extraction (vacuum cleaners, spaghetti tongs, etc.). My advice? Think of this portion of your anatomy as a one-way valve.

**Glaringly apparent lack of common sense:** Evidenced by their choice of things which shatter (e.g., glass) or splinter (e.g., baseball bats) or die (e.g., gerbils) or crawl too far up and then die (gerbils again).

**The variable:** Individual preference for the object chosen for insertion. In addition to the ones mentioned above, I've seen people who prefer cucumbers, hot dogs, candles of all sizes, vibrators, and assorted kitchen utensils (e.g., turkey basters)—uh, please don't invite me over for dinner!

■ In treating a patient with venereal disease (VD), it's important to realize that there's usually at least one other patient, since it takes two to tango. Consequently, ER physicians caution the patient to tell their sexual partner to see their physician, or come to the ER for treatment. Years ago, after treating a man for VD, I asked that he bring his sexual partner to the ER so that we could treat her. After I said that, a pained look spread over his face, and he said, "I can't do that."

For a variety of reasons, people with VD are often reluctant to divulge the name of their sex partner (or partners), so I wasn't surprised by his statement. However, I explained that he would likely contract the disease again unless she were treated, and I once more asked him to have her come in. "She would never come in on her own," he replied.

That's another objection I'm used to hearing. From my experience, people seem less embarrassed if their partner accompanies them when they're seeking treatment. So I once again asked that he bring her in. With increasing exasperation, he exclaimed, "I can't bring her to the ER!"

I asked why. He said, "They won't let her in the hospital."

Now I was puzzled. I inquired, "What do you mean they won't let her in the hospital?"

"I think there are regulations about bringing her in a hospital!" he responded. Just when I was about to ask for a clarification, he added, "Uh, she's a dog."

■ That reminds me of another story in which canine companionship was taken a bit too far. A pregnant woman came into the ER, and appeared genuinely concerned. She'd been having sex with her boyfriend and—when he was away—with his dog. Obviously ignorant of basic genetics, she wanted me to determine who was the father. I couldn't believe my ears. "Are you serious?" I asked.

"Yes. I don't want to deliver some sort of *hybrid* . . . yucch! So can you find out who got me pregnant?"

This was easy. "Well, it wasn't the German Shepherd."

■ Mike presented to the ER after sustaining a gunshot wound to one of his legs. Everything progressed normally until I routinely mentioned that I'd have to notify the police of the shooting. As soon as I said this, he pulled his pants on and began limping out of the department. I didn't have to strain my brain to figure out that something's funny here. I had the guards detain the patient while I called the police (the guards at *that* hospital were excellent, unlike some of the others mentioned in this book).

The police were very happy to finally meet Mike. He'd shot one of the officers from their department a month prior, and they had been looking for him.

■ I arrived in the room about a half-second too late. As I walked in, I noticed a puddle of fluid on the seat of the plastic chair. Since I knew that Donna had been sitting in that chair a few minutes ago, and since I knew Donna's habits, I began to warn Elizabeth. "Don't sit . . ."

She sat, but not for long. Noticing the warm liquid soaking through her dress, she rocketed upward and screamed, "Aaahhhhh! What was *that*?"

Well, technically, it was primarily water. However, the remaining constituents transformed it into a less desirable substance: urine.

Donna was a psychiatric patient who would visit the ER every few days for a variety of life-threatening and earth-shattering emergencies. Frequently, she would urinate on a chair or, when one was not available, the floor. I didn't know if she had a bladder control problem, or if her habit was a passive-aggressive means of retribution. Given that she was most apt to urinate after we failed to give in to her demands, I thought the latter explanation was most likely.

Elizabeth screamed, "What kind of a sicko would do such a thing?"

Just then I noticed Donna walking back in the room. "I forgot my magazine," she explained. She looked at Elizabeth's wet bottom and smiled. It wasn't a problem with her bladder.

■ I had to ask her. It was a standard medical question and, besides that, I was just plain curious. "Annette, why did you try killing yourself?" Her bright blue eyes now gazed into her lap, as she nervously twisted locks of her hair. No answer was immediately forthcoming, but she seemed to be formulating a response, so I remained silent. I wondered what could make a 14-year-old want to end her life. Was she having trouble with her parents? Was she pregnant? On drugs?

"My boyfriend broke up with me and . . ." She began sobbing, but sniffled twice and continued on, ". . . and he's gone and I'm afraid that no one else will want me!"

Given her stunning beauty, I imagined that she would be as popular with boys as a winning Lotto ticket would be with bankers. No one else would want her? Hadn't she ever looked into a mirror? "Annette, you're a very pretty young lady. I'm sure that you will never have any trouble finding someone to date. Furthermore, I think you're too young to worry about such a thing. Just go out with your friends and have a good time. You'll have plenty of time to date when you're older."

"But I'm fourteen!" she countered.

"That's my point," I said. "You're young. Enjoy it."

"Fourteen isn't young. My Mom was married when she was fourteen!"

I wondered what state would allow such a thing. Then I remembered the President's state of origin, and his penchant for young flesh—well, any flesh which lacked a Y chromosome. Perhaps there was a connection. I speculated as to the state.

"How did you know?"

"Oh, just a guess," I responded.

"So, if it's OK with the state, then it's OK to do, right?"

"Not necessarily. Sometimes states, in their infinite wisdom, permit people to do things under extenuating circumstances even when these things are generally not advisable."

"What's an extenuating circumstance?" she inquired.

I pulled a chair next to her bed and sat down. "Want to hear a true story?"

She looked interested. "Sure I do."

"I'll tell you about Nancy."

Nancy was a 16-year-old patient that I'd had years ago. Nancy had cystic fibrosis, a disease which sent young people to an early grave. At the time, we had no cure for the disease, and the treatments for it were abysmal. During one of her hospitalizations, Nancy's parents agreed to her marriage following her discharge from the hospital. Waiting for her to finish college—or even high school, for that matter—might be too late. Nancy was doomed to miss many years of her life, but she was determined to not miss out on everything which life had to offer. It was a good thing that she compressed her joy into such a short life, for her life was indeed short: eighteen years.

"But you're different, Annette. You're healthy. You have plenty of time in which to live life. Don't try to rush it."

"Why don't guys ask me out more often? Only one guy has wanted to be my boyfriend."

"I think they're intimidated by you. Women who are very attractive are generally not asked out as often as women who are less pretty, because most men assume that the prettiest women will turn them down."

"That makes sense. I wonder why my psychiatrist never told me that?"

"I don't know. Why don't you ask him?"

"I can't ask him," she answered.

"Why not?" I asked.

"Because he was just forced to move out of state."

Seeking a clarification, I inquired, "*Forced* to move?"

"Yes. My Dad forced him."

"Your *Dad* forced him? Why?"

"Because my Dad found out that he was my boyfriend."

# *Nothing on TV? Go to the ER . . .*

■ I'd just finished working on a husband and wife who had presented to the ER in severe pulmonary edema (i.e., their lungs were filling with fluid), triggered by exposure to carbon monoxide in their home. After they were admitted to the ICU, I wiped a thin film of sweat off my forehead as I stepped in to see the next patient.

**Dr. Pezzi:** Hi, I'm Dr. Pezzi. How may I help you?

**Patient:** I'm farting.

**Dr. Pezzi:** You're *farting*? Is anything else bothering you?

**Patient:** No, nothing else. And I'm not farting now, but I was.

**Dr. Pezzi:** Why did you come to the ER tonight?

**Patient:** Because I was farting.

**Dr. Pezzi:** But you're not passing gas now, correct?

**Patient:** No, I'm not, but I'm afraid that I will in the future.

**Dr. Pezzi:** I can assure you that it is normal to pass gas. How many times did you pass gas earlier in the day?

**Patient:** I don't know . . . four or five times, maybe.

**Dr. Pezzi:** And you came to the ER for that?

**Patient:** No, not for *that*. I came 'cause I'm afraid I'll fart again.

**Dr. Pezzi:** You will. It's normal.

**Patient:** Are you sure?

**Dr. Pezzi:** (As I gazed out the window, I stared at the glowing "Emergency" sign and wondered why a 32-year-old man would be so alarmed by flatulence.) Yes, I'm sure.

**Patient:** But isn't farting dangerous?

**Dr. Pezzi:** It's not known to be a particularly risky activity. What makes you think that it is dangerous?

**Patient:** I heard that farts can explode.

**Dr. Pezzi:** Some can, if they're directly exposed to a flame. However, this generally results only if a flame is intentionally brought into proximity with the anus at the time the gas is emitted. Besides, the resultant explosions are minuscule.

**Patient:** Are you sure I won't blow up? I'm a welder, you know.

**Dr. Pezzi:** I've never heard of a welder dying in this manner. I wouldn't worry about it.

**Patient:** Well, if I blow up and die, can I sue you?

**Dr. Pezzi:** No.

**Patient:** Why not?

**Dr. Pezzi:** Because you'd be dead.

**Patient:** Oh.

■ Working the night shift recently, I was approached by one of the nurses. She said that she had a 16-year-old female, Karen, in the triage area who gave a history of having a peptic ulcer, and the patient claimed that she had been vomiting blood and having blood in her stool. The nurse wanted to know if I would consent to treat her, since she had no parent or guardian with her to sign for treatment. In such cases, I use my best judgement of what seems to be reasonable. Obviously, in this case anyone could appreciate that she had a potentially serious medical problem. So, yes, I told the nurse, I'll treat her.

Shortly afterward, when speaking with the patient, I noticed that she gave no phone number when she was registered. Knowing the rarity of a household without a phone, I thought she was lying. I asked her why they didn't have a phone. She explained that they did, but ". . . me and my Mom and my sister talked too much, and we ran up a $900 phone bill, and my stepfather won't pay the bill, so they disconnected it." That's plausible, I thought, but I then wanted to know where her parents were. She came in with a large group of teenagers, and said she was staying with her aunt that week as she was off for spring break. I asked for the aunt's phone number. Karen said, "She doesn't have a phone." I asked about her grandparents, and she said that neither one of them had a phone, either. I told her that I would have a police car sent out to her parent's home, as I felt they should be apprised of their daughter's condition. She claimed that it was impossible to reach them, as they were at that moment on a jet bound for the Bahamas. Come on, I thought, do I have **"STUPID"** written on my forehead? I bet that there is not one family in America that can afford exotic vacations, yet can't pay their phone bill. The chance of her parents, aunt, and both grandparents having no phone was vanishingly small. Now, I *knew* she was lying, or receiving messages from Pluto—or both.

After much pressure, she finally agreed to give her father's phone number, who was living in another state. Conveniently, she gave the wrong area code, wrong exchange, and wrong number. She wasn't even *close* to the real number. After much sleuthing, we obtained her father's number. By that time, I'd called in the ER charge nurse, the head nurse of the hospital, and the local judge on-call who authorized her treatment by a court order. This little wench was jerking me around, and I was not going to give her any opportunity to come after me.

Medically, I also thought she was lying. She didn't look the slightest bit in distress, and her fashionable clothes were not stained by even a drop of blood or vomit. Once I mentioned that I wished to contact her parents, she immediately wanted to leave the ER. I wondered if she were a runaway, and decided that no reasonable person would suddenly want to leave under such circumstances, so I had the hospital guards detain her.

After examining her, and finding nothing wrong, she said that the *real* reason she was there was because she was pregnant and bleeding. I thought this was strange. It is common to have a patient tell the triage nurse and registration clerk something other than their real problem, because they may be too embarrassed to mention it to anyone other than a doctor. I've seen this occur numerous times, and it doesn't phase me the slightest bit. However, I've never had someone lead me on a wild goose chase for 45 minutes before telling me the supposed real reason they were in the ER.

Because she said she was pregnant and bleeding, I did a pelvic exam, finding no blood, no abnormalities, and nothing to suggest pregnancy. Her rectal exam didn't reveal even a trace of blood. The pelvic ultrasound was negative, showing no fetus. All of her blood tests were fine, and her pregnancy test was negative.

To make a long story short, we were eventually able to contact her mother (who was *not* on a jet flying anywhere). When her Mom came into the ER, she was furious at her daughter, saying that she has a habit of this behavior. Apparently, she likes to make up stories while out with her friends in order to garner their sympathy and to be the center of attention. *How pathetic!*

This outrageous behavior is not as uncommon as you might think. Every day, I see people claiming to have chest pain or some other potentially serious complaint, which my gut instinct tells me is not caused by any physical problem. Were it not for the fact that the United States has 96% of the lawyers in the world, I would blow off these people and save the taxpayers and insurers (ultimately, **you**) a bundle of money. However, as the game of medicine is currently practiced, doctors routinely order a bevy of tests to "prove" on paper that their clinical impression was correct.

■ Another crock case. A middle-aged woman came to the ER with her 17-year-old daughter. Both are regulars in the ER or, to put it in the vernacular of the emergency room, "frequent flyers." I knew why the Mom was there, but I decided to ask anyway. "How may I help you?"

Obviously not one to beat around the bush, she requested an injection of narcotics to treat her "migraine." Apparently vying for the world's record for the least severe migraine in history, she was in less distress than an average person with a hangnail. Needless to say, she didn't receive my vote for a narcotic. This woman is well-known to the doctors and nurses in the ER, and our consensus is that she experiences tension headaches as a result of her impending divorce. I can sympathize with the trauma of a divorce, but giving such a person a narcotic buzz is tantamount to handing them a bottle of whiskey.

On to the daughter, who complained of constant vomiting for the past hour. It doesn't take a doctor to figure out that someone who has been puking her guts out for an hour will manifest *some* signs of distress. But not this young lady, who was smiling and kidding around with her boyfriend, who was sitting next to her on the stretcher.

After a couple of hours of observation in the ER, she had experienced no further vomiting. Whenever she knew that I was looking at her, she would feign a look of distress, but her acting skills were poor. On to the coup de grâce. Just before she was to be discharged from the ER, I walked into her room and asked her how she was doing. Her countenance instantly changed from one of glee to one of agony. She flailed her arms to the side, and said in a staccato intonation reminiscent of a sheep ba-aa-aa-aa-aa-ing, ". . . barely . . .," as if she were *barely* alive. Disgusted and filled with contempt, I left the room. After walking about twenty feet, I turned around and saw the patient, laughing, giggling, smiling, and making out with her boyfriend. Pretty rapid recovery, I thought.

Psychiatrists have a label for almost every imaginable mental disorder, and most shrinks would say that this fruitcake has Munchausen syndrome, a.k.a. pathologic malingering. I prefer the term suggested by the *Merck Manual*, "hospital hobos," or in the jargon of the ER, "bullshit." Call it what you will, these people know what they are doing, and their factitious illnesses waste a bundle of money.

In this case, the tragedy is not over. This patient accused her father of touching her genitals. While no one, except the patient and her father, knows if this is true or not, the credibility of this patient is highly suspect. While she is a not-very-accomplished liar, she is a liar nonetheless. Furthermore, she fabricates stories that are intended to bring her attention and sympathy. What better way to turn on the spotlights than to allege sexual abuse?

Doctors that are duped by the Munchausenites may subject the wacky patients to needless procedures, medicine, and even surgery. Once discovered, though, Munchies pay the price of those who habitually cry wolf: no one believes them. To some, this is a pity; to others, this is a payback.

■ Let me preface this by saying that I believe women have the right to limit sexual advances. Nevertheless, it is incumbent upon women (from a pragmatic, if not a legal, standpoint) to exercise good judgement as they permit the level of intimacy to ascend. Most women have enough common sense to know when to say "no." Other women do not. Here's one who didn't.

Bertha came to the ER alleging that Steve, a guy she'd just met at a resort, attempted to have coitus with her in the resort's parking lot. This really surprised me. To begin with, it was *cold* that night, way below zero. However, alcohol can dull one's perception of cold, and Bertha had topped off her level of antifreeze in the resort's bar. I don't know how tanked Steve was, but Bertha was almost three times the legal limit of intoxication. As noted in the more professorial sections of my other books, alcohol can substantially increase a woman's testosterone level, and hence libido. This might explain why Bertha decided to leave her husband in the bar, inviting Steve to her car for some hanky-panky. Perhaps enticed by her Partonesque bosom, Steve readily accepted her amorous offer.

While French-kissing, Steve fondled her enormous breasts. Bertha didn't object. In fact, as she later told me, she enjoyed it, and decided to reciprocate the favor by performing fellatio on Steve. This was happening, mind you, about a 30-second walk from Bertha's husband. From this, I concluded that Steve and Bertha hadn't spent much time listening to Dr. Laura Schlessinger's talk-radio show.

Apparently thinking that he had been given the carte blanche green light to do as he pleased, Steve hiked her skirt and attempted intercourse. Well-pickled or not, this lady felt that such a gift was reserved for her husband alone. Since she'd give a virtual stranger a blow job in sub-zero weather in a parking lot, this struck me as a quirky truncation of morality.

But mine is not to reason why. Mine is to do an alleged rape exam—one of the least pleasant tasks in my job, made all the more so by the fact that Bertha was certain that Steve hadn't even come close to entering her. I'm not a criminologist, but I am a physician, and I know when evidence is hopelessly obfuscated. Bertha's hands, you see, had made several round trips between her and Steve's genitalia earlier in the night, when they were still friends.

About now, or perhaps a good 15 minutes ago, I'm wondering why the heck Bertha was in the ER. Steve *did* stop after Bertha nixed his plans, so I'm wondering what's the basis for her objection. Seeing that I was visibly perplexed, Bertha explained she was miffed that Steve would have the gall to even *attempt* such a thing. Bertha thought it should have been obvious that she wasn't that kind of woman. Oh yeah, that was my impression, too.

This one I'll leave for the prosecutor to sort out.

# *Fun in the snow*

■ To increase their traction, some people put studs in the tracks of their snowmobiles. As you will see, this is not always a good idea. Studding weakens the track, and weak tracks sometimes . . . well, I won't spoil your surprise.

Bob held up the back of the snowmobile while Dave revved the engine, spinning the track at 100 m.p.h. The track broke and flew backward, amputating one of Bob's legs—which was later found lodged in a tree.

■ Another hazard of studded tracks is illustrated by the following story. Scrape a cheese grater across your skin, and what do you get? Shredded skin, of course. A studded snowmobile track is analogous to a cheese grater, except that it has more power behind it (perhaps 160 horsepower). It doesn't take much of an imagination to realize that this can shred more than skin. One hapless man had the distinct misfortune of falling under the track of his snowmobile (how he managed this feat of dexterity is beyond me). His 160-horsepower cheese grater erased skin, muscle, tendons, blood vessels, nerves, bone . . . and most of his penis. I bet that his next track wasn't studded!

■ On the other end of the spectrum, a 22-year-old man came to the ER complaining that the muscles which control his right thumb were sore. He had snowmobiled for several hours that day, but had not been in an accident. (If you're not a snowmobiler, an explanation is in order. The right thumb is used to control the throttle of the snowmobile. Because snowmobile manufacturers are concerned about product liability, they typically install strong throttle return springs. The pressure required to operate the throttle is bothersome to many, if not most, snowmobilers.)

While I generally appreciate any chance to speak with a fellow snowmobiler, I was more than a little bit surprised that he felt it was necessary to come to an ER for such a problem. When I had sore muscles as a child, I wouldn't even bother to mention it to my Mom, let alone seek treatment in an emergency room. Can society afford to provide emergency room care for such trivial complaints? The answer to this primarily rhetorical question is clearly "no."

■ Steve was heading for a midnight rendezvous with his buddies at a popular gathering place for snowmobilers. Racing down a trail used to access an oil pumping station, Steve rounded a corner at an excessive speed and crashed into a tree, totaling his snowmobile. One of his legs was shattered below the knee, which prevented him from walking. Figuring that he wasn't going to be outside for long, Steve hadn't bothered to dress very warmly. As the temperature plummeted to 20 degrees below zero, he wished he had.

With a broken leg and one arm virtually paralyzed due to nerve damage, Steve was in no shape to fend for himself. To compound matters, his thinking was clouded by the booze he'd swigged just before his departure. With no survival kit and no cellular phone or transceiver, he sank into the snow for a long winter's nap.

As the morning sun peeked over the horizon, a miracle happened. Steve awoke. He—or at least most of his body—wasn't dead. Another miracle. He heard the drone of an approaching snowmobile. An oil field worker, on his morning rounds, saw Steve lying in a snow drift and brought him to the ER. Had he been in the snow for a few hours more, he would have ended up in the morgue.

■ Speaking about lying in a snow bank reminds me of the following story. This fellow wasn't a snowmobiler, but there are several elements common to some snowmobilers: excessive speed, booze, ignorance of physics, and a partial transformation into a snowman.

Mark was heading home after enriching the owner of a local tavern. With a blood alcohol level over three times the legal limit, he forgot to compensate for reduced traction caused by a raging blizzard. His new pickup truck plowed into a snow-filled ditch, ejecting him from the vehicle. This occurred in the front yard of an elderly man, who had been watching the 11 p.m. news. He looked outside to see what caused the noise. Seeing the wrecked truck, he did what any other responsible citizen would do: go to bed, thinking that someone *else* would call 911.

No one else did. When the homeowner awoke the next morning, he found a semi-solidified man lying in his ditch. Thoughtfully he now called for an ambulance.

After eight hours of blustery winds with the mercury at 25 below, Mark was lucky to be alive. Actually, when he first came into the ER, I wasn't sure if he was indeed still alive. Nevertheless, there is an axiom in emergency medicine which states that a person isn't dead until they're *warm* and dead, so we went to work.

When Mark arrived in the ER we didn't know his name, so we called him "Frosty." That was perhaps cruel, but surprisingly descriptive. His corneas (the eye's clear part) were crystallized with ice. His nose was frozen solid, as were his extremities. Had we tried to move his hands or feet, they would have shattered into pieces. They were rock-hard, as would be a steak in an extremely cold freezer. Even his abdomen had a waxy, half-frozen feeling. With plenty of TLC and lots of good ol' fashioned heat, Mark eventually made it—minus a few fingers and toes. That was truly amazing; I thought he'd lose everything beyond his mid-forearms and calves.

As amazed as I was by his recovery, I was even more amazed that the homeowner could have slept blissfully while a man spent the night in his ditch. When he was interviewed on television, he apparently realized that it wouldn't cast him in a favorable light if he were to admit that he had not called for help after seeing the accident, so he changed his story, saying that he'd discovered the crash only after he woke up in the morning. That's not what he told the paramedics, though. The viewers of that news broadcast had no reason to believe otherwise, but now you do. As Paul Harvey would say, "And now you know . . . the rest of the story."

■ And then there are people who never made it to the ER, because they were obviously dead. Such as the fellow who was snowmobiling down a road at an estimated 100 m.p.h. and struck a parked car. After such a violent impact, he wasn't even suitable to be an organ donor. Or the guy who lost control of his snowmobile while speeding and hit a tree, killing himself and his passenger, who was his 7-year-old daughter. Or the man who was run over by a car while walking down the middle of a busy 4-lane road during a blizzard at night, wearing dark clothes. Sometimes there's just no substitute for common sense.

# The indispensable ER

■ I'm truly glad this child came to the ER. Earlier in the evening, he was riding his bike until somehow—*all you product liability lawyers, pay attention now!*—the seat came off, and the seat post sheared through his scrotum, exposing his dangling testicles to the outside world. As you might imagine, this injury was accompanied by a fair amount of bleeding. The patient was too embarrassed to mention the incident to his father, and he tried to limp past his Dad in the living room on his way to bed. The Dad saw the blood-soaked pants, and brought the child to the ER.

Initially, I was reluctant to be the fix-it man for such mangled genitals. Generally, ER physicians shy away from such things, fearing an allegation that the equipment just ain't the same as it used to be. As you might imagine, the liability is enormous. Consequently, we typically refer these cases to urologists, who have plenty of experience with such surgery.

The urologist who was on-call that night thought that I'd do fine, so he asked that I do the surgery. With more than a bit of trepidation, I approached the patient who was, I'm sure, less anxious than I. Taking my time, I stitched everything back together with such precision that the nurse could not even tell where the cut was on his scrotum. I'm not much of a beer drinker, but after that I could have used one. Ahhh . . . now comes Miller® time!

■ I once worked in an area populated by a large number of people from a certain ethnic group. Suffice it to say that most Americans, given their xenophobia, are not particularly enamored with this group of people. In an attempt to prevent my untimely death, I won't name this group, but I will discuss things about them that most Americans would find peculiar.

**Their pain tolerance, or lack thereof:** Judging how much pain a person appears to be in is certainly a useful clue for a doctor (or a mother, for that matter). This diagnostic tool is virtually useless in many members of this group, unfortunately. I've had some patients, with nothing more than a sprained wrist, bellow a bloodcurdling scream that made me wonder if they were giving birth to twins and passing a kidney stone at the same time.

**Their social support system:** I'm all for a good network of friends and family to support a patient in need of TLC, but this can be overdone. *Way overdone.* On many occasions the patient would come in during the middle of the night not just with their family members, but with a few dozen people from their block, all dressed in pajamas. The ER was too small to hold all of these folks, so they would roam the hospital's hallways and even its OR's (operating rooms). OR access is restricted for sanitary reasons, but the "Do Not Enter" signs meant nothing to them.

**Their code of honor:** If they felt that their family honor was debased by a fornicating 16-year-old daughter, the father might kill the daughter. As they say, father knows best, correct?

I actually met a family in which the father had murdered his teenage daughter after she became pregnant. A few years after this happened, they brought another daughter to the ER, complaining of abdominal pain. "Oh no!" I thought, "is she pregnant?" Medically, it was a plausible explanation for all of her symptoms and signs, and I had to find out.

The nurse took me aside. Whispering into my ear, she told me of the first murder, and said that I shouldn't let any men in the family know that I was ordering a pregnancy test. Given their propensity to go wherever they darn well pleased, it was impossible to keep them away from the desk where I was writing my orders. Consequently, I employed a high-tech security measure: I shielded the paper with my hand. Annoyingly nosy, one fellow kept asking me, with an evil smile, "What are you writing, Doctor?" I gave him a verbose explanation filled with sesquipedalian (foot-long) medical words which meant nothing, both to him and me.

When the lab tests came back, I took a deep breath, and checked them. Yes, she was pregnant. I wondered what to do next.

The patient's Mom approached me. Grabbing my hand as if for both moral and physical support, she looked deeply frightened. "Tell me, Doctor, is she pregnant?" The nurse reassured me that it was safe to tell her the result. When she heard my "yes," she fell to her knees. Still holding my hand, she looked up at my face and began sobbing, begging me not to tell any of the men in her family. They'd kill the daughter, she said, and from their track record I didn't think this was a groundless concern. When I said that I would not tell the men, she—still on her knees—began kissing my hand, and thanked me over and over again. The Mom promised to "have this taken care of." She never specified what she meant by that, but I assumed she meant abortion.

Years later, as I was mulling over this event, I wondered, "What would Dr. Laura do in such a circumstance?" For those of you who don't know her, Dr. Laura Schlessinger is the host of a talk-radio show. Her specialty is delivering intelligent, pragmatic, and moralistic advice. She's incredibly witty and entertaining, to boot. I don't know what her I.Q. is, but it must be stratospheric. This lady is bright! If she were to debate Albert Einstein, I'd wish Einstein good luck. He'd need it. In addition to her other attributes, Dr. Laura is very convincing. Furthermore, she phrases things in such a way that I'm often left wondering, "Hmm . . . that makes perfect sense. Why didn't I think of that?"

So I wonder what she would do in this case. Condone the abortion, or risk the murder of the teenage girl? The latter would, of course, also kill the unborn baby. Or should the teenager be spirited off to some other part of the country to protect the life of her and her baby?

■ The triage note was succinct: "Wants something to numb back of her throat." Tough case, I thought. Must have a sore throat. I'll do a throat culture, give her some Xylocaine®, and she'll be happy. At this point, I was relieved to see a patient with a minor problem. I'd just finished taking care of several people who were critically ill, and this would be a pleasant change of pace.

Something didn't add up. People who have a sore throat sufficiently painful for them to request a topical analgesic usually look to be at least mildly uncomfortable, and Erin looked quite chipper. I introduced myself, then sat down.

"Can you give me something to numb the back of my throat?" she sprightly inquired.

I asked, "Is your throat sore?"

"No," she replied.

"Then why would you want something to numb your throat?"

"It's for my boyfriend," she explained.

"Well, if your boyfriend has a sore throat, then *he* will have to come in as a patient."

"No, his throat isn't sore, either."

I should have been an engineer after all, I mused. I could be working on things that were logical, things that made sense. This didn't. "Well, if your boyfriend's throat isn't sore, then why are you requesting this prescription?"

"You don't understand, Doctor." Evidently not. "I'm doing this *for* my boyfriend."

I was puzzled. "I thought you just said he doesn't have a sore throat."

"*He doesn't!* It's not for him to use, it's for me!"

"But you also don't have a sore throat, correct?" I wasn't puzzled, I was mystified.

"As I said, I'm doing this *for* my boyfriend. I want to numb the back of my throat . . ."

For the first time, she looked uncomfortable. To encourage her to continue, I said, "Yes?"

". . . so that I won't gag when I swallow his penis!"

■ Wendy claimed to be in labor. My cynicism, engendered by years of ER work, said otherwise. She didn't appear to be in any distress, and she didn't look pregnant. However, I'd seen a couple of women deliver babies who were so slim—from intentionally starving themselves—that they barely looked pregnant. So I had to examine her.

Sure enough, the head was already coming out. Not bothering to suction the nostrils, I completed delivery of the body. "Well, Doctor, is it a boy or a girl?" she asked.

I responded, "Um, it's a girl, alright."

She was joyous. "What should I call her? I haven't even given any thought about naming her!"

Hmm . . . that golden blonde hair, those blue eyes, that plastic body: "I think you should call her Barbie." She had "delivered" a doll.

I never ceased to be amazed at the things women insert in their vaginas. This patient was clearly mentally ill, but most vaginal foreign bodies[2] are inserted by the woman as a means of obtaining sexual gratification. In some instances, though, the patient would adamantly deny any knowledge of how "the thing got inside me." They would claim that their lover was "playing around down there" and apparently inserted something, unbeknownst to them. Maybe, but I have a hard time buying that. I've seen golf balls, Ping-Pong balls, assorted vegetables, and a silver dollar—still legal tender, I presume. I've had two or three patients with hot dogs, perhaps not surprisingly. I've discovered that these hot dogs have not fared well with the rigors of simulated intercourse; all were fragmented. I've seen broken-off douche nozzles (or whatever they're

---

[2]    *Foreign body* is a generic term used in medicine to denote the presence of an unnatural object inside the body. In the Barbie case, the term "foreign body" was doubly relevant.

called), decaying condoms and "French ticklers," long-forgotten contraceptive sponges, and . . . no, I won't say. It's too gross to mention. It's not what you're thinking; it's even worse.

■ I *will* mention the contraceptive sponge story, though. If nothing else, it illustrates an important medical principle that is germane to this topic of vaginal foreign bodies. I've seen two patients with problems attributable to such sponges. Naturally, I'll present the more interesting story.

Paula was in jail for stealing something from a local mall. Our facility had a contract with the police department to provide care for police prisoners, so when Paula developed lower abdominal pain and a fever, she was brought to see us. The female police officer who accompanied the patient stayed in the room as I performed the pelvic examination. She wasn't eager to watch, so she stood by the wall near Paula's head.

After inserting the vaginal speculum, I saw a large, white object deep within the vagina. This puzzled me for a second, then I recognized what it was. "Paula," I inquired, "do you use contraceptive sponges?"

"Yes I do. Why?"

"You have one still inside you."

"Darn!" she exclaimed. "That's the second time I've forgotten to take the thing out!"

I asked, "How long has it been in there?"

"Two weeks," she replied.

Yikes, I thought.

I grasped the sponge with an instrument and slowly withdrew it. As it left the vagina, a sudden gush of yellowish-green pus poured out of her. The smell would have nauseated a grizzly bear. Wafting toward the police officer, she sniffed once or twice, her eyes fluttered, and then she slid down the wall, unconscious. She hit the floor with a resounding thud. The patient, who couldn't see what was going on, bolted upright and began screaming, "*What happened? What happened?*" Hearing this, the nurse ran into the room to see what was going on. After we revived the officer and I calmed everyone down, I asked the nurse for some culture tubes. To make a long story short, the patient had an infection with a nasty type of bacteria, *Pseudomonas*. The infection had begun spreading through her body, and she required admission for IV (intravenous) antibiotics.

Moral of the story? Do not leave things in the vagina, since they can cause horrendous infections. If this patient had not been treated, she easily could have died. From a sponge!

■ A 72-year-old man had suffered a heart attack while having sex, but that's not terribly unusual. As Paul related the story to me, he indicated that the much younger woman with him was his lover, not his wife. Again, I wasn't surprised. Paul *was* surprised when he saw that his wife, who'd been standing by the doorway, had heard his confession.

■ I wasn't the ER physician on this case, but I was working in the ER when the patient arrived. He was at work and had been mixing paint in a large drum, using an outboard motor to do the mixing (must have been some drum!). He reached into the vat of paint for some reason, and his sleeve was caught by the outboard's propeller, which pulled him into the drum. He was literally soaked with paint on every square inch of his body. Unfortunately, the paint wasn't water-soluble, so this wasn't a quick 'n' easy cleanup. Naturally, one of the local television stations found out about this, and came to the ER for this—um, *colorful*—story.

■ The only thing worse than an out-of-control patient is an out-of-control patient who is so physically imposing that the hospital security guards and nurses refuse to even touch him. Sam was a 6'8", 275-pound mass of muscles, and I . . . well, I was no match for him, and I was cowering in fear about what I was going to do with him. The nurses were convinced that he was just crazy, a raving lunatic on a rampage. From what little history I was able to obtain, I was convinced that he was a perfectly sane person whose low blood sugar level was making him temporarily wacky. Great hypothesis, but how to test it? Clearly, we had to raise his blood sugar level. That's best done with food, but he didn't eat any of the food we gave him. He threw it back at us. I guess he *was* sane—it was hospital food, after all.

Eventually, I realized that my only viable option was to administer an injection of glucagon, a hormone which raises blood sugar. If you know what insulin does, you can think of glucagon as being the antithesis of insulin. OK, enough physiology. Back to the pragmatic question at hand: *who* was going to administer the injection?

The line of volunteers was surprisingly short. The nurses assured me that they'd sooner tender their resignations than get within ten feet of Sam. The guards were not legally entitled to deliver medical care, so they were automatically disqualified. Lucky them. That left me. Unlucky me.

As a nurse prepared the syringe of glucagon, I contemplated my fate. Would he pulverize my face, or just snap my neck? Would he jab the needle back into me? Would he throw me through the window? Or would he . . .

"Here's the syringe," the nurse interjected, "and you're the doctor. Good luck."

I thought of President Roosevelt's statement that "the only thing you have to fear is fear itself." Catchy platitude, but the Pres had obviously never met ol' Sam. I was afraid, and I was not ashamed to admit it. Fear is a conditioned reflex that quickens your reflexes, strengthens your muscles, speeds your pulse, and makes you act fast . . .

I hopped on Sam like a polecat, and plunged the needle into his arm. A second later, I jumped back. Intact. Sam gave fleeting attention to the injection, as if he'd been stung by a mosquito, then he resumed his tirade. We retreated to a comfortable distance, fifty feet or so, and just waited.

Fast-forward twenty minutes. Sam was now perfectly lucid, and he was eating the snack we gave him. "Hey, Doc, why is there food splattered on the wall?"

"Oh, we had a patient in here who wasn't very fond of our food, that's all."

"Who was that?"

"I can't tell you. Patient confidentiality, you know."

"Oh, OK."

■"That must have been *some* orgasm!" This was Paul's initial reaction as he watched his girlfriend Stacy slump backward after her climax. When he failed to awaken her, he realized that this was more than a post-orgasmic slumber, so he called 911. Coincidentally, Stacy was a nurse at our hospital, and she was only 32.

Since Stacy was comatose when she arrived in the ER, I obtained the history from her boyfriend. Paul answered "no" to the usual ER questions: booze, drugs, kinky sexual practices?

"No, Doc, she was just on top, moaning like she was really enjoying it, and then she sort of screamed and fell backward. I thought she'd had The Big O, that's all. But after I shook her and she wouldn't wake up, I thought something was wrong. Like she had a seizure or something."

A seizure would have been a comparative blessing. Stacy's coma was attributable to a cerebral hemorrhage, a type of stroke. Before the day was through, her life was over.

Lest you harbor a fear of subsequent orgasms, let me assure you—as you must already know—that reaching orgasm is not a particularly risky activity. If Stacy hadn't died as a result of her climax, she would have died the next time she strained to lift a heavy bag of trash. Considering that, she was lucky. Sexual activity, and especially orgasm, raises the pain threshold. The higher the threshold, the less subjective pain you'll experience after any given noxious stimulus. While I'm sure that Stacy had a whopper of a headache before she became unconscious, that pain must have been less intense than it otherwise would have been, had it not been preceded by an orgasm.

All of this did little to console Paul. "I killed her! I killed her with my dick."

"Not really," I said, "she just had a weak blood vessel in her brain. It was bound to rupture in the near future, anyway. Don't be so hard on yourself."

"But what do I tell her parents?"

"Well, you might want to omit a few of the details . . ."

■ Another cerebral hemorrhage story. Karl, who was 25, called his sister to say that he'd had a sudden onset of an excruciating headache, unlike anything he'd ever experienced previously. His sister, Connie, noticed that his speech was odd and that he looked to be drunk—although he never drank. She immediately brought him to the ER.

My first question was, "Does he always sound like that?" I'd never seen him before, but his speech impairment was obvious.

Connie replied, "No, just today."

As I asked her a few more questions, I noticed that he was posturing (medical lingo for odd reflexive movements of the arms and legs which indicate that really bad things are happening in the head). I quickly gave him various medications through his IV, and I intubated him (put a breathing tube into *his* breathing tube, or trachea) and placed him on a ventilator. I knew he'd sustained a cerebral hemorrhage, so I called the neurosurgeon.

"Pezzi, why the heck are you calling me? He's just going to die. It's a waste of my time to even come in," he said.

"Well, what do you want me to do with him? Take him off the ventilator, and dump him into the street?" I can be blunt, as I'm sure you've already noticed.

"Oh, shit, I've got to come in." Blah, blah, blah . . . more complaining.

While I was waiting for the neurosurgeon to arrive, I performed a few more tests. The patient was taken to surgery with the neurosurgeon still muttering under his breath about the futility of all this.

A couple of weeks passed, and I was working the day shift in the ER. I saw Connie walking in the hallway. She had come to pick up Karl, who was being discharged from the hospital. He had a mild speech problem, but was otherwise neurologically intact. I suppose I hadn't wasted the neurosurgeon's time, after all.

■ One of the standard ER questions in the evaluation of people with abdominal pain is to ask about their last meal. This often proves to be enlightening. One young lady answered, "I had watermelon, jelly beans, pickles, chips, pizza, pretzels, pop, cake, and ice cream."

I wondered if she were trying to kill herself. "Oh, and we went out for French fries, too."

■ Greg came to the ER via an ambulance, complaining of a rash on his back. He thought he should have been seen before other people in the emergency room, so he used one of the phones in the ER to call 911. Another ambulance arrived and transported him at his request to another ER, where he hoped to be seen more quickly. Only in America can such lunacy prevail.

Incidentally, every time I've seen this happen, the person has **(a)** been on welfare, *and* **(b)** had nothing which even remotely resembled an emergency. Nevertheless, given the litigiousness of our nation, the second ambulance would dutifully transport the patient to yet another ER, irrespective of whether or not such a service was necessary. Every time this happens, you can . . . *cha-ching!* . . . add another $600 to the national debt.

■ This next patient looked quite concerned, and she was on the verge of crying. "I think my hair is losing its sheen, and I'm losing weight, and my fingernails have funny ridges in them, and my skin doesn't seem to be the same color, and my bowels have been a little loose lately, and my back hurts a bit, and things taste funny, and loud noises seem to bother me more, and I'm not sleeping as well."

With a laundry list of complaints like that, you might think I wouldn't have a clue as to what was bothering her, right? Wrong. I knew *exactly* why she came into the ER. Don't ask me how I knew, because I have no idea. I just knew it.

"Ma'am, you think you have AIDS, don't you?"

She burst out crying. "*Yes!* I was afraid to say it. I've been waiting a long time to come in, because I didn't have the courage." More crying.

She'd had unprotected intercourse with a new partner, and she was afraid that she'd acquired an HIV infection. First, I reassured her that she was probably worrying about nothing. Heterosexual intercourse is not the risky Russian roulette that it is portrayed to be in the media. Next, I tested her. Sure enough, it was negative.

■ It was a little after eight on a Sunday morning, with the caffeine barely kicking in, and I was given the opportunity to be a foot surgeon. Lucky me.

Todd had been seeing a podiatrist for warts on his feet. Because his insurance covered emergency room visits, but not visits to a podiatrist, Todd decided to go to the ER for treatment of his warts. This did not strike me as a valid justification for an ER visit. However, considering the vagaries of most medical insurance policies, such behavior is relatively common. Penny wise and pound foolish, but I think the overpaid insurance executives who write the policies are more to blame than people who take advantage of such pecuniary idiosyncrasies.

Although I was not relishing the idea of wart surgery, the ER was uncommonly slow that morning, so I agreed to accommodate him. Just as he was about to remove his shoes, he froze for a second, let out a childlike scream, and then ran out of the ER. For a split second I wondered what provoked his reaction. Then I froze when I saw it, too. A man walked into the ER, unbelievably composed, holding his intestines. Thank God I'm not squeamish.

As Dave approached me, it was obvious that he was having some difficulty holding on to his bowels. They're slippery, and their attachment is rather loose. On those rare occasions when the abdominal wall is sliced open, as had happened to Dave, the intestines tend to droop out when a person is standing. A more impressive entrance to the ER is difficult to imagine.

"Hey, Doc, I've been stabbed. He sliced me right open."

Attentively, I listened as he continued on. "He told me to give him my wallet, and I told him to #µ¢* off. That's when he cut me. Think you can help me?"

"You bet," I replied, "just lie down on this stretcher." Sure beats wart surgery any day.

■ It was clear that she wasn't going to make it. Lauren was about 25, and was nearing the end of her pregnancy when she sustained a cardiac arrest. If she weren't pregnant, I would have called for the end of the code, and walked out of the room to speak with her husband. But this was different. We had one more patient to consider—her baby.

Medically, it is possible to perform an emergency C-section and revive the infant. However, that's legally known as an "operation," which requires that consent be obtained if this is feasible. Since her husband was standing just outside the door, it was indeed feasible, so I felt obligated to present this option to him. I also felt morally compelled to let him make the decision. I thought it would be unconscionably presumptuous of me to walk out and say that his wife was dead, but that I'd decided to deliver his child anyway. He didn't hesitate: don't do the C-section.

I never asked him why he'd made that decision. Was it because he didn't want to raise a child alone? Was it because the child might be a constant reminder of his departed wife? Was it because the child, at least indirectly, was likely responsible for the death of his wife? Or was it because the child, even if he had lived, would have likely sustained brain damage as a result of a lack of oxygen?

I never asked him, but he told me anyway. That was his wife, but it wasn't his child.

# On my soapbox

■ There are three classes of people who come to the ER via ambulance. First are those in legitimate need of emergency medical services. They may have been shot, stabbed, in an automobile accident, or they may be having a heart attack or some similar medical malady. The next category are the older folks who feel that their age gives them the right to call for an ambulance even if their condition is no more serious than an ingrown toenail. If they have a serious complaint, then I have no qualms with their arrival by ambulance. This is not usually the case, however. I have seen them arrive at 3 a.m. Sunday night merely because they had not yet been given a diagnosis of their condition after visiting their doctor, local specialists, and the Mayo Clinic. I'm *not* kidding! This has happened to me several times. How could anyone expect to have an emergency physician accurately diagnose a non-emergent condition, when that person's own physician could not determine the cause of their problem even when they were aided by a bevy of tests (like CAT scans, MRIs, EEGs, EMGs, etc.) and a number of consultants as well as the mecca of Medicine, the Mayo Clinic? While I can sympathize with their frustration, I think their disregard of financial considerations is inexcusable. The ambulance ride, coupled with the CYA (**c**over **y**our **@**$$) testing ordered by the ER doctor, will cost $1000 to $2000. If patients paid for medical care with their own money, they generally would not come in unless there were a worsening of their condition (which could usually be managed as well or better by their own doctor). When patients are not directly paying the bill, they often feel no compunction for expanding the national debt. Their attitude is, "I earned it!" On that account, they're wrong. Very wrong. Yes, they probably paid into the system they are now draining, but they "earned" what they are taking as much as a person who demands $100 from you just because he gave you $20. A fair trade? No, it's highway robbery. Just because it is being done by a sweet old lady doesn't make it right. The facts are simple: you will spend a significant portion of your life working to pay taxes for services that you will never receive because the money is now being spent on people who are receiving services far in excess of what they have paid for. When we are elderly, my generation will suffer disproportionately. It's not that I have no compassion for those currently retired, because I do. I simply believe they have no right to usurp more resources than they have earned, thus dooming my generation, and subsequent generations, to a miserable retirement. This intergenerational plunder is perpetuated by the reluctance of

America's elected "leaders" to face the wrath of the current generation of elderly voters. The pathetic lack of courage in these ostriches permits this problem to snowball, which virtually guarantees that the eventual solution will come about only after the carving of the Social Security pie is reordered by an internecine struggle of heretofore unseen magnitude.

The third category of people who arrive by ambulance are the scumbags. They can afford hundreds of dollars per day to buy alcohol and drugs, and have no problem finding transportation to collect their welfare check, buy drugs, beat up someone, and to find a sexual partner as oblivious to venereal disease as they are, but when it comes to getting a ride to the hospital, they think that "911" is the number for the taxi service. These people usually come in with wacky complaints—what ER doctors call "bullshit." Their complaints simply have no connection to reality. They may complain of having the worst headache of their life, yet sit comfortably on the exam table smiling, laughing, giggling, and making out with their boyfriend or girlfriend. Some headache. I've had three migraine headaches in my life, and I can tell you from personal experience that a person with a *bad* headache shows it. It's like trying to smile all the way through childbirth. Other goofs complain of having chest pain. I've had hundreds of patients, usually women aged 20 or so, come into the ER, complaining, "I be havin' this chest pain, like somebody be sittin' on my chest, and it be shootin' to my left arm, and I be short of breath, and I be sweating, and I be sick to my stomach." Neglecting her English, what she gave was a good description of cardiac chest pain[3], but I'm thinking, "This be bullshit." For CYA reasons, ER doctors order a number of tests to exclude any possible serious cause of chest pain, thus wasting another $1000 or so. And why shouldn't they? Actually, there is some justice in this, in that society is being punished (in the form of exorbitant medical expenses) for its failure to get the lawyers off the backs of the doctors. The doctors face some financial penalty for this, because they pay taxes, too (in fact, a disproportionate share, given their income). However, their personal share of this tax inflation is paltry when compared with the financial devastation that a physician faces when confronted with a lawsuit. Anyone with common sense would do the same. Even with Michigan's recently enacted caps on malpractice awards, I still face a few

---

[3]    I have noticed that people with no jobs, little education, and too much time on their hands can imagine that they have all sorts of problems. They may have heard their grandfather complaining of the same thing, and think, "Ya' know, I be feeling my chest be tight, too. I wonder if I be havin' a heart attack." If I thought about it hard enough, I suppose I could imagine that my chest is tight, too.

Incidentally, after performing hundreds of CYA evaluations of young people with chest pain, the number that have revealed unexpected findings is *zero*.

*billion* dollars of liability per year. While the risk that every patient seen by a physician will bring a suit is essentially zero, even a conservative estimate of the potential financial risk faced by a physician working in a busy ER will show that he faces several hundred million dollars of liability per year. You might be shocked to find out how often records are subpoenaed by attorneys looking for a case. This usually goes nowhere, because doctors in America have learned that the CYA game is an integral aspect of medicine. This testing often does nothing to benefit the patient, and his outcome is the same if the doctor had done nothing to evaluate him. But what would happen to the hapless doctor who did not have the correct tests documented to prove that his clinical impression was correct? He'd be sued so often that he couldn't afford to eat stale bread on sale. Thus, Mr. and Mrs. America, we doctors are forced to choose between bankrupting the country, or facing bankruptcy ourselves. It's a tough choice, and you know how it is turning out.

The medical malpractice system benefits very few people, and harms everyone else. It has driven a wedge between you and your doctor. It has increased your taxes. It has increased the cost of all goods and services. It raises your insurance premiums (not only for your health insurance, but for your car, home, boat, snowmobile, motorcycle, etc.). It forces you to wait longer to see a physician (playing the CYA game takes time, you know). It forces you to undergo countless tests and procedures needlessly. It encourages expansion of the government and of the insurance industry; does this benefit you? *NO*. People are no better off in terms of their health than they were 40 years ago, when medical malpractice lawsuits were as rare as dodo birds. Did doctors give any less attention to their patients then because they were not scared out of their minds by the prospect of a lawsuit? If you don't know the answer to that question, think about this—when was the last time your doctor made a house call?

Years ago, doctors didn't worry about being sued, but they certainly did not ignore their patients. Even as an ER doctor, I have a few patients that I trust implicitly; we have developed a mutual trust and I can treat them as I would a member of my family: if something needs to be done, I'll do it, but I don't order needless CYA tests. Unfortunately, those people are in the minority. Many people today walk around with a chip on their shoulder, and it doesn't take a genius to realize that they would sue over a cup of bad coffee if they could get away with it. Those people are CYAed to the max, and if they are actually so obnoxious (or idiotic!) as to mention "attorney" or "lawsuit," they may as well forget about bringing a lawsuit because the doctor will generally do such a superb job of CYAing that no lawyer would touch the case. Malpractice attorneys are like burglars in that they look for easy targets. Make it tough for a burglar to break into your home, and he will look elsewhere. Make it tough for the lawyer to cast some doubt on your medical treatment, and he will find an easier target to support his resort in Vail.

If you think all of my bitching about malpractice lawsuits is simply a one-sided attempt to help myself and my colleagues, you're wrong. In what must be one of the ultimate ironies, medical malpractice has actually *helped* most physicians[4]. Except for the few physicians whose personal assets have been pillaged by the system when a judgement exceeded their malpractice coverage, most physicians have reaped a huge financial benefit from the current system. How so? Without the worry and attendant CYA engendered by malpractice suits, the amount of tests and procedures that I do would plummet, along with my income. Financially, I'm certain that I am far better off under the current system, because I'm smart enough to play the game. But does this help you? No, it doesn't. I am rallying against the current malpractice system because of its nefarious effect on society. Frankly, I don't care if my medical income is reduced by 70%, as I have many other means in which I can make money. In short, I'm doing this for you, not myself.

■ I'll never forget that day. The paramedic radioed in that he would be bringing some injured patients to the ER. One patient had a dislocated hip, and her daughter's legs were paralyzed. Another car had crossed the centerline of the road, and struck their car head-on. As so often happens, the at-fault driver wasn't injured. He hadn't been drinking, but he was "intellectually challenged"—or whatever the politically correct term happens to be this week.

The orthopedic resident quickly reduced (i.e., corrected) the Mom's hip dislocation, but the daughter was another story. Tiffany was ten, and from the paramedic's original report I knew that she had sustained a severe injury to her mid-thoracic spinal cord. Sure enough, everything below that level was paralyzed and numb.

---

4       If you have read much of this book, you will probably be struck by a similar irony: while I am adamantly opposed to the general concept of welfare, I (and other emergency physicians) have actually profited from it. Sure, we have paid considerably more in taxes as a result of it, but our income *with it* is disproportionately greater than what we would make *without it*. Because the government requires ERs to treat all people regardless of their ability to pay, the number of people treated in emergency rooms without insurance (and, hence, less likely to pay for their care) would rise astronomically if welfare were eliminated. Welfare-sponsored insurance programs do not reimburse providers as well as private insurance companies, but *some* money is certainly better than *no* money.

I had the nurses prepare to administer anti-inflammatory steroids intravenously as soon as she arrived, as that was the current standard of practice. We gave the steroids, but they made no difference. She was still paralyzed. I wasn't surprised. You may be, though. Some of the things we do in medicine are done not so much for the patient, but to ward off a potential lawsuit. Had I not given the steroids, Tiffany's outcome would have been no different, but she could have sued me for a million dollars—and won. I thought that she was entitled to compensation for her injury, but why sue *me*? I didn't cause the accident. Why not sue the responsible party? But such lawsuits are about draining the deep pocket, not about seeking justice. And I knew that if Tiffany's care wasn't 100% perfect, I'd pay as if I were 100% responsible for the accident.

So I gave her perfect care, according to an expert orthopedic surgeon who later reviewed the case. She would still spend her life in a wheelchair. She would never dance again. She might never get married—and if she did, she could never have a normal sex life.[5] In short, her life was horrendously marred, if not ruined. Who could she sue? She could sue the driver who caused the accident, but his sheltered workshop wages wouldn't make for much of a settlement. If there were justice in this world, she should be able to sue whatever state official issued a driver's license to the impaired fellow. But there isn't justice in this world; the politicians have seen to that.

---

[5]     She might, however, be able to experience orgasms. As detailed in my book *Fascinating Sex Secrets*, due out in late 1998, it has been discovered that women may be able to experience orgasms via an alternate pathway. Incidentally, this applies to any woman, not just those who are paralyzed.

# *Love, lust, & sundry propositions*

■ A young man had come into the ER with his girlfriend for suturing of a cut he had on one of his hands. The procedure was uneventful, but the conversation during the repair was not what I had expected. His girlfriend, Kris, asked, "How much money do you make?" Not wanting to answer that question, I merely smiled. She then speculated, "I bet you make $20 an hour, don't you!"

One of our star nurses, Larry, happened to be in the room at the time, and replied, "He makes more than that!"

Her eyes now gleaming, she said, "Wow!" and continued her speculation. "I bet that you make $40 an hour, don't you?" Again, I smiled and said nothing.

Larry piped in, "Higher!"

Reaching an apoplectic frenzy, Kris blurted out, "I want to date you!" Mind you, this conversation was held in front of her boyfriend! I felt sorry for him, as he seemed to be a very nice young man and he certainly didn't deserve anyone as shallow as her. I kept wondering what she would have said—*or done*—if I had told her how much I really make.

■ When I began working at the hospital in Flint, I lived in Livonia, which was 63 miles away. Consequently, I would usually stay in Flint while I worked for a few days, and then go home to enjoy some time off. One of my first routines upon arriving home was, not surprisingly, listening to my answering machine. One message was brief, but to the point, saying in a seductive female voice obviously tinged by alcohol, "You treated me in the emergency room, and now I want you to treat *me!*" I racked my brain trying to think who it might have been, not because I would have done anything with her, but simply out of curiosity. Given the number of people that I see in the ER, it was difficult to associate her voice (the alcohol didn't help, either) with any patient that I had recently treated.

■ Some women are more immediate in their approach. A couple of years ago, while wearing a green scrub suit and standing at the nursing desk writing orders, a patient asked one of the staff members a question about me. In a loud voice she inquired, "Is the guy in the green pants a Doctor?" When told that I was, she exclaimed, "He's a cute little thing, isn't he?" For some reason, people tend to perceive me as being small. This is baffling to me, since I'm 5' 8½" (and don't forget that extra ½"!) tall, which is very close to the average height of a man.

Several months later, I went into an examination room and asked a patient how she felt. She paused briefly, smiled, and said, "The more I look at you, the better I feel!" Another young lady, lying on a stretcher in one of the hallways, blurted out, "There's that cute Dr. Pezzi again! I saw you a few months ago. Remember me?" Such comments surprise me, because I never thought that my appearance warranted such encomium. I suppose there is something about a "doctor's coat" that makes a man more appealing.

■ Others are not so subtle. A beautiful 16-year-old once asked me to a boat party. Perhaps having spent too much of my life staring at books and playing with transistors, I had no idea what a boat party was, so I asked her, "Ah, what's a boat party?" She explained, "It's where we get together on a boat at night *and drink!*" Cognizant that I am somewhat of a nerd, I was certain that I—28 years old at the time—would have very little in common with a bunch of drunk teenagers. It would also make for quite a scandal; I can hear it on the TV, "Doctor parties with group of intoxicated teens. Story at 11." I passed.

■ On the other end of the age spectrum, a 67-year-old lady being seen for chest pain asked me, "What are you doing when you get off work?" As I tend to have a thick skull sometimes, I asked her, "Why do you want to know?" In an ardent and almost hormonally-induced ebullience she proclaimed, "*So we can party together!*" At least she, and the 16-year-old mentioned above, were nice enough in their approach; I can't say the same for the following person.

■ Working the afternoon shift a few years ago, I asked the other doctor working with me if he would mind seeing a patient. This patient had made a few prefatory remarks toward me which led me to the conclusion that my encounter with her would not be on a very professional level. Although the administrators at my hospital might find this hard to believe, I do try to steer clear of trouble, but the other Doc wouldn't help me out. "No, you go see her, Kevin. She's *cute!* She likes you!"

The patient didn't waste any time. "What's your phone number, Doc?"

Feigning stupidity, I asked, "Do you mean the number of the emergency department?"

"No, I want your *home* number!"

Trying to reply in a geez-why-would-anyone-want-that? tone of voice, I said, "Why?"

Leaning forward, smiling, and rolling her hips slightly, she explained, "Because I want to date you!"

Still acting stupid, I inquired, "Why would you want to date *me*?"

She was blunt, and without batting an eye she said, "Because I want to make love to you!" Having met this person about 5 minutes ago, I knew she was not one to waste time. Without any encouragement on my part, and perhaps in an attempt to entice me, she then went on to describe in graphic detail other things she wanted to do to me. And then, in a tone of voice that suggested that her next comment would not conflict in any way with what she had just offered, she continued, "Oh, I think I may have AIDS. Can you check me for AIDS while I'm here?" I wasn't surprised.

■ Julia was another devotee of the direct approach. I'd seen Julia in the ER recently, and she apparently liked me, because she came to give me the key to her apartment. I wasn't working on the day she returned, so she gave the key to the on-duty ER doctor, asking him to forward the key to me. This piqued his interest, and he began chatting with her. It didn't take long for the doc to realize that this person was deranged, so he committed her to the psychiatric ward. Another great romance bites the dust.

■ "I don't want to get married again, I just want to sleep with you." Typical guy-talk, eh? Nope. This was uttered by a former patient when she called me at home. Obviously, being bashful was not one of her problems. As the conversation progressed, I began to think that she may have taken the "Reach out and touch someone" AT&T slogan just a bit too far. Somehow, I had a difficult time picturing ol' Pez transmogrified into a stud. Perhaps a tad less implausible than Mr. Rogers moonlighting as a male escort, but shocking nonetheless. This being impossibly at odds with my self-image, I declined her generous offer—uh, offer*s*.

■ *Ouch!* A prominent, though inebriated, local business owner came to the ER with a cut near an elbow. She was in her mid-30s and strikingly attractive. Successful, intelligent, beautiful—and a *woman*—well, she seemed out of place in an emergency room. Nonetheless, she made herself right at home. Since her cut was on the back of her arm, I had her lie in the prone position, with her injured arm extended along her side. Halfway through the suturing, she began rubbing my upper thigh. This was not exactly on my list of the "10 most likely things to happen during my shift," and I was literally frozen, unable to speak or move. A few seconds later, she glommed onto a nearby portion of my anatomy. Then she squeezed.

*Hard*. Reflexively, I jumped backward, still mute. Her head, which had been resting on a pillow, turned toward me. She smiled sensuously, and purred that her exploration was unintentional. *Sure*.

■ On the opposite end of the sweetness scale was Angie. Everyone has had certain experiences in life that are cherished memories; this is one of mine. The hospital in which I work is a teaching hospital, meaning that we train physicians, nurses, and paramedics. Angie was enrolled in the paramedic program. I often have the paramedic students follow me around so that they get involved in interactions with patients, and so that I can teach them.

On her first day in the ER, which was very busy, Angie accompanied me on my rounds. After a few hours, I made a comment about wishing that I could eat, which I could not do because the ER was too busy to allow me to go to the cafeteria. Angie then disappeared for several minutes. Walking into my office, I was astounded! The lights were off, and the room was illuminated by a flashlight that Angie had directed at the ceiling, to simulate a candle. One of the tables in the room had been cleared off, covered with a table cloth. Angie had china, silverware, napkins, salt and pepper shakers, and a smorgasbord of food covering the table. She also had a bouquet of fresh flowers, placed in a vase that she had improvised from the ER paraphernalia. Music played softly in the background. *Gulp*. I was so taken by what Angie had done, I probably would have asked her to marry me, if she were older.

■ Speaking of marriage . . . It began uneventfully enough. The ER was packed full of patients, most of whom clung tenuously to life. It was past midnight and, as usual, I was the only ER physician working. While writing orders at the nursing station, I glanced up to find a *stunningly* beautiful woman walking by. When I saw the wrist band which indicated she was a patient, I was more thrilled than I would have been if I'd won the Lotto. That meant I'd have a chance to talk to her. Just one problem, though. My *other* patients. They had come to the ER on a pell-mell journey toward death, and it was my job to save them. Accomplishing that feat would take a few hours.

Patiently, she waited. Introducing myself, I felt discombobulated by her whiplash-inducing beauty. Her face was gorgeous at rest, but when she'd talk or smile, it moved in an indescribably delicious dance, sending waves of rapture through my increasingly apoplectic mind. I'd never before, or since, seen a face move that way—a way that, until then, I would have thought to be impossible.

To her cat, though, that face was not a work of art to be treasured, but a launching pad of escape from a feline nightmare. Lynn's cat had been sleeping on her pillow, when he suddenly awoke in terror. Bolting for the confines of safety, his claws had shredded a 5-inch patch of skin on the side of Lynn's face. I'd seen plenty of cat scratches before, but never anything this deep. Undoing that damage would require more than an hour of meticulous work, not enough time for my discombobulation to dissipate, but sufficient time to flirt. I'd offered to remove her stitches myself, and she accepted. Sure, it was primarily a ruse to see her again, but I also deemed it to be medically necessary. Lynn's personal physician was not noted for his surgical skill, and the thought of him clumsily attempting to remove the tiny stitches that I'd so carefully placed left me cringing.

A few days passed, and it was time for suture removal. I drove to her home and removed the stitches. A professional success, but a personal disappointment. I was almost ready to leave, and she hadn't reciprocated any interest. Being realistic about my chances of dating a goddess, this hardly surprised me. Then she said that she wanted to see my house. This could mean that she had an interest in architecture, or me. I was hoping for the latter.

I was right. Much later on, she told me that her interest in my home was simply *her* ruse to see me again. Necessarily coy, I thought at the time.

Months passed. We had been dating, and somewhere along the way we'd decided to get married. We never did, though. If you guessed *why* we broke up, you'd probably be correct.

■ The other former patient that I'd dated came to the ER after being involved in an automobile accident. Annette wasn't nearly as beautiful as Lynn, but she was cuter—if that makes any sense—and she exuded sex appeal. Not in a stuck-up sort of way, but in a friendly, oh-so-huggable, chemical attraction which made my hormones rage. It didn't hurt that she came wrapped in a body which seemed to be the personification of lust.

We didn't waste much time. On our first date, we raced go-carts, then went to a movie theater. I didn't see much of the movie, because she was sitting on my lap and—better yet—facing me. If her passionate kissing was at all indicative of her passion for other things, I was in for a real treat. I was in for something, but it wasn't a treat.

Next stop: dinner at a restaurant. I doubt that she would have batted an eye if I'd suggested going to a motel instead, but I'm a bit more old-fashioned (and circumspect) in such matters than you might imagine.

To tell you the truth, it didn't even cross my mind at the time. Remind me to have my testosterone level checked, will you?

Back to the restaurant. Halfway through dinner, and totally out of the blue, she brought up the subject of marriage. Trying to paraphrase her eloquence, or lack thereof, simply wouldn't do it justice. So, let's turn the dial on the time machine, and hear it verbatim. As Walter Cronkite used to say, ". . . and you are there."

**Annette:** You know, I'll marry you, Kevin.

**Me** (surprised by such a premature revelation)**:** Uh, you want to marry me?

**Annette:** Yes, and I don't care what you look like, either.

What she lacked in tact, she made up in honesty. Translating her last comment, it became, "Yes, Kevin, I'll marry you. You're ugly, but you have more than enough money for me to overlook that. I'm a gold digger in too big of a hurry to bother with any pretense of being adroit. So, bub, it's your money for my bod. Fair trade?" No, Annette, it's not.

▪ You meet someone. You really like them, and you wonder just how much they like you. You'll find out, some day, somehow. But when? Well, it never crossed my mind that I'd find out while doing a physical exam in the ER. I'd been dating Lisa for a few weeks, and we'd had a good time together. She seemed to be quite interested in me, but she didn't exhibit any romantic feelings. I'll just bide my time, I thought.

On one of our dates, Lisa told me about her back problems. She was hoping to recover some damages as a result of her back injury, but her attorney said that she would need some medical verification. She suggested that I examine her in the ER, so that she would have an official record. I was too dumb to realize that I was being suckered, so I agreed to examine her.

After I completed the exhaustive documentation of her history and physical, Lisa had another request: would I examine her breasts? I *was* interested in her breasts, but I didn't want to *examine* them. And certainly not in an emergency room. Why was she asking me to do that? Whatever she wanted, even if it was *just* a breast exam, I knew that this could mean but one thing for me—that she had no romantic interest.

"Well, will you?" she asked again.

I realized that I'd been silent. Didn't she know that this was an odd request for a supposed friend, even if he was a doctor? Didn't she realize how awkward it must be to be dumped during the middle of an ER visit? But the game was over, and I'd lost. No use groveling. "OK, I'll do a breast exam. I'll have a nurse step in as a chaperone."

I never saw her again.

■ As I came on for the night shift to relieve Ben, he gave me a synopsis of the patients he was turning over to me. "Oh, you'll like the next patient," he beamed.

"Why is that?" I dryly inquired.

"She's a stewardess. Absolutely beautiful. And *stacked!*" He motioned with his cupped hands in front of his chest, as if I didn't know what "stacked" meant.

"What's she in here with?" I asked.

"Chest pain. You lucky guy. She's single; have a good time."

"Ah, she's probably dating a pilot. They make as much money as we do, and nobody sues them, even when they plow a 747 into the side of a mountain on a sunny day. Why is it that only doctors are personally sued?"

"Pezzi, people hate doctors. Haven't you figured that one out yet?"

Her EKG, chest x-ray, and blood tests were unremarkable. Darn. I was hoping for an easy out. But, with no obvious diagnosis, I was forced to do what I dreaded most: I had to examine her—and her chest. Oh, I know what you're thinking . . . horny young doctor can't wait to cop a feel of the beautiful bombshell. Personally, I'd rather examine an 88-year-old great-grandmother. Then, if I have to do a breast exam, no one would question the legitimacy of it. I'd never do any exam unless it was indicated, but I can appreciate how patients might think otherwise. And, with a bod like that, I was afraid the stewardess would think I was just having a bit of titillation. No pun intended.

I was correct. As I was palpating her chest wall (which *was* tender, thus providing the diagnostic clues), she commented, "I bet you like your job."

I searched for an answer that was sufficiently ambiguous. "You might be surprised."

■ And now, as the epilogue in this confession session, I have to mention that I once kissed a patient *on the lips* in the emergency room. True, she was about 90 years old. I can't recall what was her presenting complaint, but the reason she was in the ER boiled down to one thing: she was lonely. Her husband had passed away a few decades earlier, and her remaining family seemed disinterested. Sad. There wasn't anything *medical* that I could do for her, so we talked. At some point during our conversation, I kissed her. I can't give you any cerebral explanation for the kiss, because there wasn't any conscious thought behind it. It just seemed as natural as hugging a child with a boo-boo. To say that the kiss lifted her spirits is an understatement. Afterwards, she was smiling, cheerful, and content. She felt that *someone* cared, and I did. Some people are genuinely likeable, and that she was. I suppose I could have given her a prolix explanation that I cared, but somehow it wouldn't have been the same.

■ These days, one of the problems with young women is that they often don't look like *young* women—they look like sexually mature, above-the-age-of-consent women. Chalk it up to the many chemicals in our environment which act as synthetic estrogens, or whatever. Regardless of its causation, it can create some nightmarish problems for men who think with their wrong head.

Jennifer was brought to the ER by her parents, a state social worker (I'd never actually seen one before), and an entourage of police officers. I guessed that I'd soon be filling out a lot of paperwork. I was correct. Jennifer had been dating Harry, who was 31. Jennifer was, well, stunning. With a bod like that, she could have been a Miss America. Who'd have thought she was only 14?

Her parents were upset by this, but couldn't do much about it. They'd ground her, but she would find a way to see him. One day, as Jennifer was staying with her grandparents, Harry stopped by. He took Jennifer on an unauthorized date, to an unauthorized motel, for some unauthorized fun. Now her parents had him. They immediately called the police, and whisked her to the ER.

Jennifer seemed as reticent as Monica Lewinsky, as she was reluctant to say anything which might incriminate her partner. Eventually, she said that Harry had engaged in "no improper sexual behavior" with her. Gee-whiz, with lingo like that, I thought she was being coached by White House lawyers.

OK, he'd engaged in "no improper sexual behavior" with her. But did he have *sex* with her? Turns out that he did. Fancy phrases are often contrived as a means of obscuring the truth.

■ As Stan and Mindy walked into the ER, I guessed from their attire that they had attended the senior prom. Noticing the blood on Mindy's gown, I surmised that this was the reason for the ER visit. I was correct on both counts.

Having never attended a prom, I have only secondhand, anecdotal reports of what goes on during and after such an event. Suffice it to say that losing one's virginity after the prom is not a rare occurrence. Indeed, Stan and Mindy had succumbed to their youthful passion and consummated their long-term three-week relationship. While most women manage to lose their virginity without a subsequent visit to the ER, most women do not have to contend with Stan or someone like him. More about him in a minute.

Initially, I guessed that the source of the blood was from the ruptured hymen. Sure enough, the hymen was bleeding I found as I performed the pelvic examination. But that wasn't all. The vagina itself was torn and bleeding. I wondered how that had happened.

**Mindy:** Oh, God, it really hurt when he put it in me.

**Dr. Pezzi:** I can imagine . . .

**Mindy:** I've never had sex before, Doctor, but this isn't the first time I've seen a penis. But I've never seen one so huge! I mean, I didn't think they came that big.

Neither did I. To make a long story short, Stan wanted my medical opinion on whether or not he was a freak of nature. His terminology, not mine. A caring physician would be amiss not to euphemize such an aberrancy in a more sensitive manner. Having been trained at Wayne State, I thought I was ready for this.

Let me digress for a minute. At Wayne State University's School of Medicine, we were shown dozens of pornographic (OK, *highly* pornographic) films as part of the curriculum. The rationale for such an unusual academic inclusion, we were told, was so that we would not react in disgust if a patient revealed sexual proclivities that were, well, strange. By exposing us to every imaginable sexual practice, they hoped to desensitize us so that we could just deal with the medical issues, leaving judgement about such practices to God, or perhaps to Jerry Springer and his audience.

As Stan dropped his trousers, my eyebrows reflexively raised.

**Stan:** What do you think, Doctor?

**Dr. Pezzi:** Well, Stan, it's certainly a very large penis.

**Stan:** Do you think I'll be able to have a normal sex life—you know, without hurting women?

**Dr. Pezzi:** That depends upon your partner. If she has a small vagina, it will be uncomfortable for her.

And dangerous, too. Knowing how sensitive young people can be, I didn't want to give him a complex about his penis. In truth, I should have answered that he would be unlikely to find a human female who would be a suitable match for him, size wise. Although I have seen thousands of penises, I'd never seen one which was even remotely similar in size to that of Stan. The next largest penis was, I'm sure, at least four times smaller in terms of volume. I bet Stan's Mom rinsed their dishes well when he was a kid . . . but that's a story I'll leave for some of my other books.

■ After Dawn worked her last shift at our hospital, she went to a bar, ostensibly to celebrate. I'm not sure how much celebrating she did, but she certainly did a lot of drinking. Medically speaking, she was plastered. That was apparently only the first phase of what she had in mind. The next phase of her plan was to register as a patient in the ER, which she did. Legally, this just gave her justification for being in the emergency room, in spite of her unruly behavior—which was the ultimate objective.

You might think that Dawn would have started bitching about the hospital or something like that, but that's not what she had in mind. She liked the hospital, and one nurse in particular. *That's* why she was there. With her inhibitions at an all-time low thanks to the booze, she now felt comfortable announcing to the world—or at least everyone within earshot—that she had the hots for Bill, one of the male nurses in the ER. Not coincidentally, Bill was working at the time.

Since her loud proclamations would have earned a "XXX" rating, I can't give you a verbatim account of what she said. However, she expressed her fondness for Bill's body, indicating that she wished for a certain part of his anatomy to be repeatedly thrust into her body. She wanted some steamy sex, and she wanted it *right now*, on the ER stretcher. Apparently thinking that Bill would actually grant her wish, she removed her clothes, spread her legs, and made other preparations for their forthcoming tryst.

Understandably, this drew plenty of attention in the ER. It was like a soap opera, minus the commercials. When one of the patients (who was being seen for a psychiatric reason) saw that Bill wasn't rushing to pleasure Dawn, he volunteered to assuage her libidinous desires. "Hey, baby, if he won't bang you, *I will*."

An elderly patient looked over at me and said, "Has everyone gone nuts in here?" I felt compelled to give her a candid answer. "Yes, they have. Welcome to the ER!"

# The ER as a dirtball magnet

First, a word of introduction. Emergency room personnel use the terms "dirtball" and "scumbag" synonymously. While both are admittedly pejorative appellations, they are appended only to individuals who richly deserve such a characterization. It is believed that they are derived from the old Latin words "dirtballitus" and "scumbagitus," which referred to individuals whose personal hygiene was subhuman, on the order of a pig. In deference to their modern social connotations, these terms are not applied to people who *cannot* attend to their hygienic requirements. Thus, a person who is paralyzed and unkempt is simply a person in need of a bath, not a dirtball. Furthermore, usage of these terms has been broadened, and they are now commonly applied to individuals with a variety of disgusting and reprehensible traits.

■ When I worked in the ER, I had an opportunity to meet a wide variety of people. I met some of the best people in the world, and some of the worst. George was in the latter group. An admitted drug dealer, he bragged about how much money he made. He made more money than an average orthopedic surgeon—and he, of course, did not pay any taxes on his income. To compound matters, George was on public assistance. Now for his bad traits. George had one of the most obnoxious personalities of all time. He was not just despicable, he reveled in it. He found glory in recounting how he had severely beaten people, yet had always managed to escape before the police came.

When I saw this character in the ER, he initiated our conversation by stating that he would not pay the ER bill. Punctuating this statement with a smile so vile that the Grinch would be jealous of it, he luxuriated about how his "official" near-zero income made him immune to the obligation to pay his bills. That attitude is quite prevalent among the recipients of welfare[6]. As a physician who was often made privy to the personal secrets

---

[6]    Believe it or not, but I'm not totally opposed to welfare/Medicaid. There are some decent, normal people who *temporarily* receive such assistance in times of need, and there are people with profound handicaps who have a genuine need for long-term aid. Unfortunately, the original intent of such legislation has been warped so that simple laziness is often the only qualifying condition that "justifies" the receipt of public assistance. My beef with such people is that they consider employment, public responsibility, and community service to be concepts that are irrelevant to them. They want *you* to get up at 6 a.m., drive to your job, work your butt off all day long, drive home, pay your bills, flop into bed exhausted, and do the same thing day

in and day out until you're 65—all so they can leech off you, getting up whenever they darn well feel like it, sit on their fat you-know-what all day long, smoking cigarettes that were purchased with *your* money (thus inducing disease that *you* will pay for), overeating food that *you* bought (in other countries, poverty often results in starvation; in America, there is a greater-than-average chance of finding obesity in people on the rolls of welfare—pun intended), and then they and their politicians have the gall to suggest that *you're not doing enough for them*, that you're not giving your "fair share." ***Bull!*** Like insatiable pirates, the greed of such people is limitless. You are already giving far more than you should—it's the career leeches on welfare that need to enroll in Responsibility 101 and start contributing to society. How often do you see the professionally unemployed people taking the initiative to volunteer their services to the community? In addition to providing about $70,000 worth of free medical care each year to poor people, I keep clean several hundred feet of street in my neighborhood (and I've even washed it, after the utility company covered it with mud), I pick up trash in my neighborhood (if people in the ghetto did this, there wouldn't be a ghetto!), I've helped a disabled veteran do housework, and I have three jobs! It's a good bet that the welfare folks have a lot more free time than I to do such community work. But they don't. What's their excuse? Laziness. For them, it's "me, me, me, give me, give me, give me." A quid pro quo? A return? Some gratitude? Ha! Suggest that, and they will respond with contemptuous umbrage. There's a sign in the Rocky Mountain National Park which aptly summarizes the welfare problem: "Please do not feed the squirrels. If you feed the squirrels, they'll become overweight and prone to disease. Their population will grow, and they'll lose their ability to forage for food on their own. They will expect you to feed them and will attack you if you don't. They'll become like little welfare recipients, and you wouldn't want to do this to them."

Even when I look at some of the more compassionate aspects of welfare, such as the assistance of mothers and children with deadbeat fathers, it is obvious that there is often an unconscionable lack of responsibility and judgement on the part of these mothers that created their predicament. In watching nature programs on television, I am impressed by how females in other species are selective in their choice of a mate. In species in which the male plays an integral role in providing for the offspring, there are elaborate mating rituals which ensure that only supportive males are allowed to mate. Why should it be any different for humans? Most mothers are understandably picky in their choice of a mate, but this is often an extraneous concept to women on welfare, who view the financial support of their children as something that is deservedly dumped onto the backs of the taxpayers. I don't agree with that. If a man is irresponsible, women shouldn't sleep with him. If they have children anyway, they should get a job and support their kids. Can't do it, the job doesn't pay enough? Baloney. I'm tired of that pathetic excuse. My Mom raised three children without my Dad in the 1960s, when women's pay was disproportionately lower than it is today. She had no college degree—just a lot of gumption. As Dr. Laura Schlessinger says, "If you're going to take on the accouterments of adulthood, take on the responsibilities of adulthood." Another eloquent Dr. Laura quote that's pertinent to this subject: "Even birds have enough brains to make a nest before laying an egg." It's funny that many humans have yet to master this concept. Not coincidentally, this irresponsible behavior is primarily present in countries in which people know that the government will be there to bail them out.

We coddle them. We give them free food, shelter, and medical care. We put spending money in their pockets. And what do they do for you? Statistically, the welfare folks, and their progeny supported directly and indirectly by you, are more apt to possess a host of undesirable traits, all of which have the potential to make you absolutely miserable. Certainly, *not* all of them are bad people, but they're *more likely* than an employed person to be a thorn to society, in addition to being an obvious drain on society. They have a higher rate of alcoholism, and are more likely to smash into your car while driving, thus turning your family outing into a nightmare, and your daughter into a paraplegic. (The thought-control police might object to such an "offensive" asseveration, but it's true. I've seen children permanently

**54**

of my patients, I learned that most of them on welfare have sources of income that they conveniently forgot to report to the government. Being officially poor, they consider financial obligations to be a concept that is irrelevant to them. Ignoring their bills and taxes made them able to afford things that are far beyond the means of most Americans. If an ER doctor were to turn these people in, they would get a lawyer to sue the doctor for malpractice, saying that the doctor violated the "sacred" confidentiality of

---

paralyzed by people whose life, car, and gas money was sponsored by the welfare system. Funny, I've never seen a teacher or a barber or a janitor paralyze anybody. Now then, what's more offensive—harsh, *but factual*, words, or a kid who is destined to spend 75 years in a wheelchair?) They are more likely to engage in a variety of crimes. They shoplift, so you pay more for the goods you purchase. They make your visit into the city a hair-raising, pulse-pounding, gut-wrenching horror, making you wonder if you will reach your car before someone sticks a knife in your belly. They burglarize your home, steal your car, and bash in the skull of your Dad. Hyperbole? Hardly! It happened to my Dad. His lifeless body was then dumped into a swamp, and left to rot in the muck. They are more likely to abuse drugs, which indirectly contributes to crime and the spread of pestilence. They clog up emergency rooms, making you wait, and wait, *and wait*. They reproduce at a disproportionately high rate, making more welfare recipients for you to support. They warp the political and economic milieu of America, turning it from a dynamic land where success is rewarded to a place in which it is punished, subjecting productive people to punitive taxation and mindless scorn. Having too much time on their hands, and being more inclined to devalue life, they are more likely to commit malicious "pranks." When I was training in Detroit, a scumbag dropped a bowling ball off a freeway overpass, which shattered the windshield of a passing vehicle. The ball hit the driver (an ophthalmologist) in the head, splitting his skull and spraying his brains over the interior of the car, and onto his wife and daughter. It's enough to make you vomit. On another occasion during my stint in Detroit, I was studying at the medical school library with another fellow, who made the mistake of leaving a few minutes before me. We both walked down the same street, but he had the misfortune of flushing out a miscreant who was lurking in an alley. The dirtbag stabbed the fellow to death, and took his keys and wallet. His address was listed on his driver's license, which prompted the wicked leech to pay a visit to the victim's apartment. There, he found the man's wife, who he then raped and murdered. And, to top it off, he found their 9-month-old baby, who was stabbed repeatedly, and beaten into a lifeless pulp. Kill the baby? What's the kid going to do—finger the criminal in a lineup? The perpetrator of this savagery is unbelievably evil, and the legal system in this country is pathetically unable to mete out a commensurate punishment. This man, and others of his ilk, don't deserve to live. While it is not possible to abort such human trash beforehand, it *is* possible to encourage behavior that will minimize the likelihood of similar barbarity. The answer is simple: we must stop rewarding people for sitting on their butt, and send them off to work. The need to work forces marginally adaptive people to yield to the need to conform—or else. In other words, shape up or ship out. Since we're speaking of *working* to *survive*, those who don't feel like working will not be around to pulverize babies. In past times, people were arrested for vagrancy, having "no visible means of support." Viewed from a modern perspective, such an action might appear to be unduly harsh, but it makes a lot of sense. To survive, people must obtain resources either legitimately—via work, or illegitimately—via crime. Vagrancy thus becomes a useful marker for ferreting out criminal activity that might be otherwise difficult to discover. Let's get people to work, and into the mainstream of society. Let's stop electing the "something for nothing" politicians who cater to the welfare crowd. Let's stop looking for magical, pie in the sky solutions to the vexing problem of crime, and instead look to an answer that is so obvious it is being overlooked: work. Work. It's good for you. Welfare is not.

the physician-patient relationship. The confidentiality doctrine was not intended to be an inviolate shield to protect criminals, but the rampant aggressiveness of "personal injury" attorneys has cowered physicians into an extreme reluctance to report illegal activity.

■ Some dirtbags assume they can tell a physician anything, and that he won't *dare* turn them in. Wrong. Take the case of Frank, for example. Frank came to the ER for repair of a cut on his hand. Being the inquisitive fellow that I am, I asked him how he had received the cut. He said that it had somehow happened while he was stabbing his girlfriend. "Oh, really?" I thought. His cut was minor, and my thoughts immediately turned to his girlfriend. I wondered if she were lying somewhere bleeding to death, so I asked Frank if he had bothered to call for an ambulance to assist her. Not only had he not called, he said, he refused to tell me where she was so that I could send an ambulance to help her. After pleading with him to cooperate, it became obvious that he wanted her to die. He felt that if the only eyewitness to the crime was dead, and the doctor was afraid to report the crime, that he would be a free man. "Oh, really?" I thought. I was determined to see that his girlfriend got help, and determined to see that he would not get off scot-free. I called 911 and had police sent to the ER. The officers "encouraged" him to reveal the location of his bleeding girlfriend. After I repaired his cut, he was handcuffed and taken to jail. Touché. Just another Saturday night in good ol' Flint, Michigan.

■ I think emergency physicians have a moral and ethical obligation to be part detective. There would be no need for this if every patient we faced were an honest, law-abiding person, but that's unfortunately not always true. By paying attention to my gut feelings about certain people or situations, I've ferreted out murderers, attempted murderers, drug dealers, pimps, con artists, thieves, and people trying to perpetrate a variety of frauds and other crimes. This hasn't done much to increase my popularity among the criminal set, many of whom would undoubtedly like to shoot me. It also hasn't done much to increase my popularity with hospital administrators, some of whom would also like to shoot me. Administrators view the incarceration of a patient as a lost opportunity for revenue. If their trip to the ER lands them in prison, there's a fat chance they'll pay their hospital bill, right?

I'm certainly no Sherlock Holmes, but—given the intelligence of most criminals—I certainly didn't need to be so gifted. Here's a typical case.

Ted and Bob walked into the ER, and Ted registered as a patient. When I quickly scanned his chart before going to see him, I noticed that Ted gave no phone number or local address, and he had no driver's license or social security card. No credit cards, either. Uh, excuse me, isn't this the 20th century?

I listened intently to Ted's story, even though I thought it was BS. He claimed to be from another state (another planet was more like it), and was in the area to erect a gas station canopy. I knew of no local stations that were under construction, and I didn't believe this skill was so esoteric that there was a need to import out-of-state workers to have it performed. And where is his crane—in his trunk? Or was he planning on renting one from Cranes-R-Us? Furthermore, he was traveling by car from another state, and he had no driver's license with him? *Sure*, I believe that!

Ted claimed to have back pain and he requested a narcotic injection, and a prescription for more narcotics. Having seen many of his ilk with even better acting skills, I was a tad less than surprised by his request. When I explained that I wasn't going to comply, he began yelling at me. Bad move.

I walked to the registration clerk's office and asked her to call the local police to check out these two characters. She made the call, and a dispatch was made over the police radio for a cruiser to stop by the ER. That's when the fun began. The clerk was a police radio aficionado, and her trusty police scanner picked up the dispatch. Bob, who was sitting in the adjacent waiting room, heard this dispatch and decided that he and Ted would hightail it out of there before the police arrived. Does this spell g-u-i-l-t-y or what?

The police cruiser pulled into the ER parking lot just as Bob and Ted were pulling out. I indicated to the officer that they had just left, and he followed in hot pursuit. Eventually, he caught up with them and pulled them over. In the car they had numerous license plates, fake ID's, driver's licenses, and—curiously—discharge instructions from an emergency room about an hour north of us, which Ted had visited earlier in the evening. He'd also received a prescription for narcotics. Funny, he'd neglected to include these trivial details in his medical history. As it turned out, Bob was an armed robber. Great guys, eh?

Of all the characters in the story, the dumbest was not Ted or Bob. The dumbest one was the ER physician at the other hospital, who was duped by a pathetically inept pair of bunglers. These guys were transparent with a capital "T" . . . how could he not have known? I suspect that he may have known, but succumbed to administrative pressure to accede to patients, no matter what. This "give 'em what they want" motto is suitable for a fast-food restaurant, not an emergency room.

■ I believe that emergency physicians have an obligation to protect society members from patients in other ways, too. One particularly revolting case comes to mind.

I was working the afternoon shift along with another ER physician. One of his patients was a rather hardheaded man with AIDS. This fellow refused to stay put on his stretcher. Time after time, he'd unhook his IV (intravenous line), and then stroll through the hallways of the hospital, dripping blood from his dangling IV line. Notwithstanding the esthetic drawbacks to this hallway hemorrhaging, I was aghast at its potential lethality. Kids have a habit of touching things which interest them, and I was afraid that some 3-year-old would put his hands in the blood, and then into his mouth, nose, or eyes. Seeing that I was apoplectic, the nurses went after the patient and brought him back to the ER. They'd restart his IV, and everything would be OK for a few minutes. Then the patient would walk off again. Realizing that this patient was an inveterate wanderlust, I told the guards to restrain him to the bed.

"Can't do that, Doc."

"What do you mean you can't do that?" I demanded.

"It's against his rights," this legal scholar opined.

"I'm not particularly concerned with his rights at the moment. What I'm concerned about is the people he is endangering by dripping his blood throughout the hallways. He's infected with HIV, and his blood is deadly! Some child could touch the blood and infect himself—and could die as a result!"

"Yeah, but there ain't nobody forcin' the kids to touch his blood, so we ain't gonna tie him down."

Although I was convinced at this point that there were chipmunks with higher IQ's, I continued to try to reason with the guards. "Look at all these children!" I said, pointing to the kids in the hallway.

"They their parent's responsibility. Ain't your's, and ain't mine."

Such erudition. "Parents cannot watch their children every second. A kid might touch the blood before the parent even knew it was there!"

"Look, as I been tellin' you, it ain't your problem, so leave it alone!"

Disgusted with his insolence, I warned, "I'm not going to debate this matter with you. I'm in charge of the ER now, and I'm ordering you to restrain that patient!"

The guard's jaw tightened. He looked like he wanted to slug me, but he turned and walked away. But not after the patient. I returned to the emergency department, and asked the nurses to restrain him. "We'll put him back in bed, but we won't restrain him."

The same argument ensued, although it was conducted on a much higher level. They presented their interpretation of the relevant hospital policy and applicable laws, but I felt that such theoretical concerns about administrative repercussions were overshadowed by the manifest danger that this patient presented to the hospital's visitors. Let the legal chips fall where they may, I implored. I couldn't imagine that a judge or anyone else imbued with an ounce of common sense would have faulted my decision to restrain this person. Still, the nurses refused. They restarted his IV, and left the room. Have we become a nation in which laws and regulations supersede common sense?

I tried reasoning with the patient. Didn't work. I tried bribing him. Didn't work, either. "I likes walkin' around the hospital," he declared.

I once more explained the dangerous situation he was creating for others, but this didn't seem to move him. "Hey, I've got AIDS. I don't care nothin' about nobody else. I hopes that everybody gets it and dies with me."

I closed the door. Pointing my finger at him, I said, "Look you jerk, you're going to stay put in *this* bed. You've exposed hundreds of people to the HIV virus, and you obviously don't give a shit about that. If you try leaving once more, I'll glue you to that bed with Super Glue!"

"You can'ts do that!" he said in his unpolished English. "You do that, and I be suin' you!"

"That's funny," I said, "you're concerned about *your* rights, but you don't care about anyone else."

"Why should I?" he asked contemptuously.

"For your own self-interest, if nothing else. If you walk out there again, I'll have you arrested for attempted murder. You'll go to jail, not some nice comfy hospital bed. I'm not going to tell you again. I've got patients to take care of, and I'm tired of wasting my time in here! Got it?"

Apparently he did. He didn't walk off again.

■ To conclude this section on dirtballs, let's look at a case in which that term was particularly appropriate. Vernon's presenting complaint was such that I was compelled to examine his genitals. After I peeled off his tattered yellowish-gray underwear, I noted that his scrotum was covered by numerous dirtballs. These appeared to be small spherical accretions of dirt, dead skin, skin oil, underwear lint, and heaven-knows-what-else.

This was too much for me to bear. Until this point, I'd put up with a variety of noxious insults to my senses, with nary a complaint. One fellow's back smelled so bad that when he sat up on the stretcher, the smell from his back caused me to actually vomit in the ER (how a *back* could stink so badly is beyond me). Did I complain about that? Nope. But I'd reached my breaking point now. I asked him, "By any chance, are you allergic to soap and water?"

He responded, "No, why do you ask?"

I said, "Because it's apparent that neither of those substances has contacted your skin in years!" The nurse was even more direct, chiming in, "You're disgusting! I'm not even touching you until you take a shower!"

Vernon apparently felt the need to explain his personal hygiene, or lack thereof. From his explanation, it was clear that he reveled in the disgust evinced by prostitutes whom he'd hired to perform oral sex.

The nurse was livid. "*That's it!* I don't care if you *do* take a shower—I'm still not touching you!" With that, she stormed out of the room.

I thought everyone's mother had warned them to always wear clean underwear. Vernon never got the message, though.

# *How* **not** *to win friends & influence people*

■ I suppose it is human nature for a person to be more inclined to attack someone they think they will never see again. This explains why people sometimes react violently when they are driving around someone who they feel has wronged them, and it explains why people are more apt to vent their anger at an ER doctor than their own physician. Irene, the irate grandmother, comes to mind. Earlier in the day, she took her granddaughter to her pediatrician, and was given a topical medication to treat a diaper rash. She applied the medicine once and, lo and behold, the rash was—*surprise?*—still there! Around midnight, Irene came into the ER along with her granddaughter, who she claimed was in excruciating pain. As I walked into the room, I noted two things: 1) the child was sleeping soundly, and 2) Irene was mad—I mean *M-A-D!* Steam was pouring out of her ears and nostrils, and her face was contorted with rage. "I applied the medicine once, and the rash isn't gone!"

It is perhaps not unreasonable to question the validity of her bewilderment. After all, she's made one application, and 98% of the medicine is still in the tube. If one application could effect a cure, why would the doctor be so wasteful as to prescribe enough for a few weeks of treatment? To me, this point seems to lie in the realm of common sense, and does not qualify as an esoteric medical concept. But, with one application and no cure in sight, Irene was furious. "Someone is going to pay for this," she fumed. Did she call the pediatrician? No, that would be too logical. Instead, she popped into the ER. I explained that the resolution of this rash would require healing, and that there was no way for skin to heal so rapidly. I also deftly suggested that the treatment will take more than one application of the medicine. A few tips later, she was anything but pacified. With all of the charm of an enraged pit bull, she *screamed*, "I want this rash cured, and I want it cured now!" Her anger was both misdirected and unfounded, and I wondered how anyone could get through 60 years of life and still be so stupefied by something so basic. My efforts to reason with her were fruitless; she yanked the sleeping child off the examination table, and stormed out of the ER, cursing and threatening all the way. A Dale Carnegie graduate, she was not.

■ ER patients who are abusive scumbags usually blithely assume that meting out abuse is a one-way street, with them as the givers, and the helpless ER staff as the takers, whose hands are tied by professionalism, thus preventing them from retaliation. Oh, if they only knew! Most ER personnel I've met are furious about the abuse they receive, and some *will* retaliate.

I won't bore you with the routine tit-for-tat acts, such as stuffing a sock into the mouth of a scumbag with a penchant for spitting on people. Well, maybe I will bore you with that one. One of the best ER assistants I ever knew was fired after it was discovered that he put a sock into the mouth of one of the all-time scumbag stars who frequented that ER. The scumbag spat on him, and he retaliated. Can you blame him? Sure, there are more professional ways of dealing with such abuse, such as the oxygen mask technique that I prefer (put an oxygen mask on a spitting patient, and the spit ends up where it belongs: on the face of the patient), but I think most people would not tolerate such a personal affront. Spit into the face of a police officer or, for that matter, a truck driver or a carpenter, and see if they calmly wipe the spit off and walk away. Notwithstanding the civil libertarians who might be abhorred by such an act, I think that anyone who spits on a police officer *should* be punished—and I don't mean in the pansy courts, either. Police officers have a tough, stressful, and dangerous job. Through my work in the ER, I've gained an understanding and appreciation of their work, and I give police officers the same level of respect that I give to my physician colleagues. A police officer is also, in a sense, a symbolic embodiment of the good in society. As a member of society, I *don't* want scumbags and riffraff desecrating officers.

Now, let's return to the case of the sock-stuffing ER assistant. He was paid $7 per hour to work his butt off at all hours of the day and night, weekends and holidays included. He has put up with vicious, profane, threatening, and violent ER patients for years. He's been punched. He's been kicked. He's been urinated on. He's been threatened in countless ways. He's been cut, scratched, and had his hair pulled. He's had his glasses broken. He's had people vomit on him—*intentionally*. He's put up with this crap for years. Sniveling hospital administrators have done nothing to mitigate the decline in his morale, invariably siding with the patient in any such dispute. "The patient is always right, the patient is always right . . ." they chant in their elegant offices, as they lean back in their $1000 leather chairs. With such abuse, and so little support, is it any wonder that, sooner or later, a person will retaliate?

I once worked in the ER of a city that had more than its share of violent people. With alarming frequency, one of these jerks would beat up the entire ER staff, and all of the hospital security guards. Someone would dial 911, and we'd be rescued by the police. Would the offender be taken to jail? *Heck no!* Take him to jail, so that the taxpayers can pay for his

62

food, lodging, medical care[7], and legal expenses? So that he can be on the street in another six months, ready for another round of ER bashing? *No way!* They'd take the scumbag into an alley, beat the $#!+ out of him, and leave him to lick his own wounds. Now, that's Biblical justice. Funny, we never had any repeat offenders. If the scumbags ever came into the ER again, they never tried to start Round #2. Do you think the courts could have done better? Check their rates of recidivism, and it will be clear what type of justice is more effective.

Before I delve into the next revelation, I want to make one thing *perfectly clear*: it is of no use to subpoena me before a Grand Jury to wring out my testimony on who said this, because I honestly can't remember who did. Maybe they were just kidding . . . and maybe they were serious, dead serious. As a further prefatory remark, I should also note that it *wasn't* me who said these things. My way of dealing with abusive scumbags, as if you haven't already noticed, is to lambaste them in print. The pen is mightier than the sword, right?

Well, not everyone agrees with that. I've heard more than a few ER personnel muse over the injection of various nasty things[8] into the veins of hated patients. I'm not talking about *whoops!-too-much-potassium, your-heart-has-stopped* instant murder, but rather an injection from a syringe filled with enough germs to provide a case-of-the-year presentation at an Infectious Disease Grand Rounds. The most recent twist—such an apropos word in this context, isn't it?—on this theme is to assassinate someone by injecting HIV. *Yikes!* No more yelling at the nurse, right? Deep down, I think that the people who said such things were just blowing off steam. In any one 4-year term, about half the people say they'd like to shoot the President, but this rarely happens. And who hasn't wanted to punch their boss in the nose? Just blowing off steam, right? Let's hope so!

■ Now that I'm on the subject of revenge, I'll include a story which still mystifies me.

Years ago, I was looking through some books in the ER office when I came upon a letter which was stuffed in one of the books. I didn't recognize the handwriting, and it was signed "Your Bro."—presumably for "Your Brother." The letter told a twisted tale of retribution which, with a

---

[7]     I suppose we should give him a Bugs Bunny Band-Aid®, too!

[8]     Occasionally, this problem occurs inadvertently by prior contamination of multi-use drug vials. Your best defense against this problem is to insist that all injectable medicines given to you be taken from a new vial. This may not increase your popularity with the nurses, but you can seek their favor by buying them pizza or flowers.

bit of Hollywood embellishment, could form the basis for a captivating movie. I've long since forgotten some of the details, but I have a vivid recall of the basic elements.

The writer, who I'll call John, said that one of his friends was a physician who was sued by a woman—for what, I don't know, but it was apparently on behalf of a relative. Neither the physician or the woman were specifically named, so I'll call them Todd and Kim for clarity. The case was settled out of court, and Todd was angry that this black mark on his otherwise perfect record might hinder his appointment to the faculty at a prestigious medical school. Furthermore, Todd knew that his wealthy parents were aghast at seeing him named in the newspaper as a defendant in a malpractice trial. So, Todd decided to even the score. He enlisted the aid of an old friend who was now a private investigator, and dug into Kim's personal life. He discovered that she was single but anxious to get married, and he learned what she was looking for in a partner. He decided to become that partner.

Todd began hanging out at one of Kim's favorite nightclubs, and Kim was drawn to this handsome, magnetic stranger who was everything she was looking for in a mate. (Apparently the two had never met during the course of the legal proceedings, which is not uncommon.) Todd said that he was a pilot for a major airline, and since he was a *private* pilot, he knew enough pilot lingo to make this seem plausible.

After several months of dating, Todd convinced Kim to transfer her investments to a different company. Since Todd seemed to have a lot of money, she assumed that he knew what he was doing in the stock market. Eventually, Kim began pressuring Todd to get married. Todd said he loved her, but that he wasn't physically drawn to her. She was slim, but Todd—bless his heart—liked big women . . . *really* big women. That explained, in Kim's mind, why he had never tried to sleep with her. But, given the plethora of restaurants serving mega-calorie meals, gaining weight was not a problem for Kim. If that's what Todd wanted, that's what she would become. Fat.

A couple of hundred pounds later, Todd assumed that she was adequately ballooned, so he dropped out of her life. She panicked at the loss of her ersatz boyfriend, and she panicked when she learned that she had lost almost all of her money in the stock market. Todd thought that he'd exacted a sweet revenge: she was virtually penniless, and about 320 pounds. End of story? Not yet.

Along with her weight gain came various health problems, which led to her hospitalization. Unfortunately for Todd, he was the physician accepting new admissions on the day Kim was admitted. She immediately recognized him, and when she learned his *real* name, she quickly put 2 and 2 together, realizing that she'd been targeted for revenge. Her plans for revenge were brought to an abrupt halt by Todd's suicide. Thinking that she had nothing to gain but personal humiliation, she quietly let the matter drop. The last John (the letter writer) knew, she had lost most of the weight, but was still broke, and still single.

■ My gut feeling told me that I'd see her again. The cause of the problem, I suspected, was that I'd been my usual nice self. For people used to gruff, disinterested, uncaring doctors, seeing a nice doctor might make them think that something more was going on. In this case, there certainly was none of that. At least on my part. But as I left her room, she said something (I can't recall her exact words) to the effect of, "Hey, am I really something, or what?" With no response from me, she said, "You like me, don't you?" I smiled and walked out, saying nothing more. While Terry was an attractive woman in her twenties, I was not drawn toward her. Lucky for me.

A few weeks later, Terry came to the ER via ambulance, complaining of knee pain. Accompanying Terry was a somewhat older friend, Dawn. As Terry was brought in, she waved to me and smiled, as if we were old friends. I suspected that she'd come in to continue flirting. I was partially correct.

When I went to see Terry, she wanted to talk about "us," not her knee. I soon regretted the way I'd truncated our first meeting with a smile. I realized the smile, at least in Terry's mind, had affirmed her suspicion that I was hot for her. At the time, I thought the smile was a semi-clever means of being disingenuously vague about my true feelings. I now realized I should have been more frank with her, but the ER was too busy for me to consider such a luxury.

And the ER was even busier tonight. Terry's conversation was centered around our inevitable relationship and blissful future together, not her knee. Much to her obvious chagrin, I was not reciprocating any romantic interest. I wanted to talk about her knee—*silly me!* It took her a while to realize that this was the only thing I wanted to discuss, and when she realized this her countenance and demeanor took a 180-degree turn. They say that hell hath no fury like a woman scorned, and whoever "they" are, they're correct. Her pretty, smiling, happy face transformed into a scowling embodiment of hate and anger. Her once sweet, alluring speech was replaced by a rough, screaming voice, peppered with profanity. She demanded an injection of narcotics, which I didn't think was indicated in this case since she originally appeared to be in no pain, and since she was originally more than a trifle reluctant to even talk about her knee. Yet, the screaming and yelling continued. Trying to give her the benefit of the doubt, I offered to give her an injection of a non-narcotic pain reliever which had no euphoric (pleasant buzz) effect. This ticked her off even more, and she refused it, still clamoring for the narcotic. As I left to see other patients, Dawn began pestering me about the narcotic shot. The ruckus that Terry and Dawn were raising was seriously interfering with the functioning of the ER, so I stepped in to see Terry once more. I briefly but courteously explained that I was willing to give her something, but I didn't believe that a narcotic was the appropriate choice in this case. This attempted appeasement flopped. Terry and her friend began bitterly complaining once more, yelling so loudly that they could be heard throughout the emergency room. After venting their spleens for another hour or so, they walked out, much to the relief of the other patients in the ER.

■ Lori was a truly gorgeous 16-year-old on her first date, and they were heading for Big Boy® or some similar house of fine cuisine. En route, they were involved in a serious car accident, and Lori's face was shredded by numerous cuts. To complicate matters, some parts of her face were so mangled that sewing her together was more of an artistic exercise than it was a surgical task. While I've had a lot of practice putting people back together again after such tragedies, I knew she would have scars, both physical and emotional. It seemed so sad. To be on her first date, and to have had such a bad accident. To add insult to injury, her date for the evening—who was barely injured—did not stay with her in the ER. I'd bet that was their last date together.

# The Twilight Zone

- A slim, well-dressed, attractive lady came to the ER, announcing, "I'm here to deliver my baby." Oddly, she didn't *look* pregnant. The triage nurse asked her how far along she was in her pregnancy, and she responded, "Two years." Somehow, I guessed that this would not turn out to be a routine ER visit. She claimed that she was impregnated in Russia by artificial insemination two years ago. Oh, those zany Ruskies, what are they up to now? When asked why she had not yet delivered the baby, she responded, "Because no one *told me* to deliver it." Makes sense to me! However, she felt that the time had come for her delivery, and she insisted upon being placed on a stretcher immediately. This accomplished, she began groaning, panting, contracting, and pushing as if she were truly in labor, until the "delivery" was completed. "My baby, I've finally delivered my baby!" Delivery, yes. Baby, no. Lying on the stretcher, between her legs, was a pile of . . . feces.

- Another strange obstetrical story. This happened when I was in medical school, not the ER, but I doubt you will mind that it doesn't qualify as an "ER story."

During my OB (obstetrics) training, I was an observer when a particularly large woman delivered her baby. The only memorable thing about that delivery was that the stirrups weren't strong enough to support the weight of her legs, and they collapsed repeatedly. The staff would reposition the stirrups and tighten their clamps, but her legs came crashing down again and again. With every collapse, the patient would let out a squeal. Such a high-pitched, bird-like sound seemed to be an incongruous emanation from such a large person.

A week later, this same woman was readmitted to the hospital. I assumed that she had some problem or complication related to her recent delivery. I was correct—they'd left another baby inside! Fortunately, this twin born a week later (I wonder if they would celebrate the same birthday?) was fine. Given the thick envelope of fat which shielded her womb, her obstetrician had been unable to detect the second child by any means, including ultrasound. Yikes!

- It's Saturday morning, and my shift was almost over. Glancing up at my next patient, I was surprised by the appearance of her face, which was shredded by dozens of crisscrossing razor cuts. However, the patient had another surprise in store for me.

The 18-year-old Julie had been at a party a few hours ago. Another woman, jealous of her beauty, decided to level the playing field by cutting her face. Julie claimed there had seen a single assailant, but I found it difficult to believe that one person could inflict so much damage without assistance. After a single cut, most people would beat a hasty retreat or, since this was in Detroit, pull out their Uzi®.

After I'd been suturing for a while, Julie said, "Hey, Doc, what's taking so long?" I explained that I was being very meticulous, so her scars would be as inconspicuous as possible. I expected her reply to reflect gratitude, or at least understanding. Not quite. "I want you to hurry up!" Again, I explained I was taking my time so that she would obtain a good result. My "logic" was not persuasive. She continued, "It's *Saturday* morning."

I didn't understand what she was getting at, so I said, "So?"

Julie, marching to the tune of her own drummer, said, "It's Saturday morning. I've got to get out of here—*the cartoons are on!*"

■ As the nurse walked over to me, she rolled her eyes up and said, "Hey, Pez, want to see a real wacko? He says that he's hearing people talking inside his mouth. What a lunatic!"

I wasn't so sure that this was an imaginary problem. This happened to me once when, as a teenager, my mouth began receiving the radio broadcast from WJR in Detroit. Until then, I would have said that anyone with such a claim had a few screws loose. As bizarre as this phenomenon may seem, there's actually a physical explanation for it that is easy to understand (at least if you have an electronics background). In certain circumstances, parts of the mouth can act as a crystal radio and thus emanate sound, albeit not very *much* sound. Here's an excerpt on this subject that's taken from my book, *Fascinating Health Secrets*:

This tip may seem to be unrelated to health, unless this phenomenon occurs to you, in which case this info will erase your self-doubts and restore your sanity. If your teeth have ever received radio broadcasts, you might think that you've entered *The Twilight Zone*, or that you're a candidate for psychiatric evaluation. If this has happened to you, my professional words of advice are: chill out. You're not insane. You're not imagining things. You haven't been drinking too much—well, maybe you have, but it didn't cause this problem! Seriously, though, it *is* possible to receive radio broadcasts in teeth that have metallic fillings. Given the increasing popularity of the new nonmetallic composite fillings, I am afraid that the next generation will grow up without having experienced this supernatural occurrence. Pity. To become a biological Walkman®

(*Toothman®?*) is one of the most mysterious, mind-expanding marvels of life. Bereft of Quaaludes® and dental radio reception, can the eternal search for the true meaning of life ever be fulfilled?

Tuning into reality once more, let's examine a "spec sheet" on dental radios:

## S.O.N.Y. *(Supernatural Oral Nighttime Yabber)* AM RADIO

| | |
|---|---|
| **Reception** | AM band only (if you think that you're receiving an FM station, you are—in psychological terms—"out of tune") |
| **Aural mode** | Monophonic |
| **Antenna** | Integral metallic dental filling or appliance |
| **Operation** | Generally perceptible only at night in a *quiet* room |
| **Speaker** | Built-in water-resistant tweeter |
| **Power output** | Miniscule (well, look at the bright side—no one will ask you to "turn it down" and you won't go deaf!) |
| **Power supply** | Demodulated electromagnetic waves (think of it as a crystal radio) |
| **Frequency response** | Crummy |
| **Total harmonic distortion** | Ditto |
| **Weight** | Depends upon your dentist |
| **Accessories** | None |

■ It's been a crazy week in the ER, and I still can't believe it. The leadoff batter in the weekly cavalcade of insanity was an alleged murderer who wanted me to believe his chest pains earned him the right to sleep in the hospital, instead of in the jail. Patients who are prisoners complain of chest pain so often I'm certain this trick is taught to them in jail by fellow inmates, or by their attorneys.

After evaluation, I decided I'd rather not sleep under the same roof as a man, it is said, who makes the Boston Strangler seem as gentle as a masseuse, so I sent him back to the slammer. After the usual threats about suing me, he said something that made my spine shiver: he claimed that a motorcycle gang was coming to town to avenge the injustice of his incarceration. The timing of that threat led me to believe I was on his revenge list. Such a threat may seem hollow, but this guy was a few chromosomes shy of being biologically capable of civil behavior, and I'm sure his buddies were no more genetically endowed. Desperate for some means of self-defense, I decided to bring a can of pepper spray with me to work the next day. I'm not sure if pepper spray has been tested for effectiveness against enraged motorcycle gangs, but I felt it would be better to spray them than to shoot them; the latter option would convert them from "biker" to "patient"[9].

My next patient was a woman who felt the best way to clean a wound was to give it a whirlpool treatment in her bathroom toilet. Even though she assured me her toilet was very clean, it did little to dispel my conviction that this lady was nuts.

The next ER patient gave new meaning to the term "utter revulsion." He complained that worms were boring into his legs. Skip the psychiatric consult, because this was no imaginary problem. There, squirming in some sort of annelid nirvana, were a dozen or so worms, burrowing with hell-bent fury straight into his legs. Pinching myself to ascertain that I wasn't having a nightmare about some Japanese horror movie, I did what any doctor on the verge of regurgitation would do: I told the *nurses* to pull the worms out! Consulting various specialists in wormology convinced me that my suspicion was right—these worms were behaving abnormally. Given that they were in an ER, though, I suppose that I shouldn't have been surprised. I suspected these worms were hatched in the soil around the septic tank of a junkie, and the PCP-, LSD-, and amphetamine residues warped the little minds of the worms, inducing a psychotic frenzy of aggression that transcended, by several phyla, the usual worm targets.

About now, I'm hoping for a patient with a run-of-the-mill ankle sprain, sore throat, heart attack, or gunshot wound. Well, I got my wish—*sort of*—for a patient with an ankle injury. Nurses have often told me that I tend to attract patients with strange problems, and many patients have said they feel as if they can tell me anything. Some have said they told me things they've never told their own doctor, or even spouse! The next fellow would have had a tough time concealing his problem, though, even if he decided I wasn't so easy to confide in. Buried in one of his ankles were several 3½" 16d nails. The nails didn't just penetrate the skin—they went deep into the bone. He looked as if he had been attacked by a cross between a porcupine and a mad carpenter, and I was at a loss to understand how this had happened, so I asked him. In a voice so casual that it might suggest this was an everyday occurrence, and with a why-would-anyone-ask-such-a-silly-question tone, he said, "I did it." Oh. My curiosity got the best of me, and I asked why. "My psychiatrist said he

---

[9]    Incidentally, the bikers *did* show up, "Nazi"-style helmets and all. They didn't find me—I found them.

wouldn't see me today, so I got mad."[10] The bit about the psychiatrist didn't surprise me.

A few x-rays later, I had an audience crowding around me as I viewed the radiographs. The x-ray technician had brought the patient's old x-rays to the ER, so I put them on the viewing box. His last ER visit was about a year prior, at which time he had hammered an even greater number of nails into his left knee. Hoping to terminate this annual self-mutilation event, I suggested to the patient that he use a plastic toy hammer and nails if an overwhelming urge for body hammering should develop in the future. I was somewhat surprised by his ready acceptance of this idea. "I bet it would hurt less. Why didn't I think of that?" Beats me.

After such a run of patients, I was debating whether this was a full moon, or a once-per-millennium celestial syzygy, or just what the nurses refer to as a "Pezzi night." My answer came with the next patient. To borrow—and modify—a phrase from a popular television game show, "Wacky patient #5, *come on down!*" The patient was a 23-year-old man who came to the ER with his ex-fiancée. His reason for visiting the emergency room? He wanted me to convince his ex-fiancée, who had just dumped him, that she should still marry him. Fortunately, I'd never before seen this fellow, or his former fiancée. Even after years of ER work, seeing a variety of oddballs, I was stunned by such a request. True, he was on welfare. Recipients of public assistance often present with unusual problems, but this request was in a class by itself[11]. Until this time, I thought I'd seen everything there was to see in an ER, but the patients on this shift were proving me wrong. Regaining my composure, I asked, "What makes you think that I can convince her to marry you?" He responded, "Because doctors are smart, I thought you'd be able to think of something that would change her mind." I thought to myself, "Buddy, I'm not *that* smart!" A full moon? A syzygy? A Pezzi night? I'll answer (d), all of the above.

■ I was doing my best to keep from laughing. A 20-year-old welfare recipient was complaining about how no one would hire him. To his credit, he *was* looking for work, but I found it hard to believe that he was mystified by his string of rejections. His hair was woven into a couple of straight, skinny foot-long projections which looked more like antennae than devil's horns. Whenever he would move, they would bob back and

---

[10]     Another psychiatric patient had a more direct way of expressing his dissatisfaction. When his psychiatrist refused to see him, he drove his car through the psychiatrist's office.

[11]     Doesn't it just give you a warm glow inside to know that your tax dollars paid for this "emergency"?

forth, giving him the credibility of a cartoon character. Had they been hiring at McDonald's® on the planet Mars, he would have been in luck.

■ If you're over 40, you may recall the old documentaries narrated by Walter Cronkite. At the culmination of the introduction, Cronkite would say in his inimitable style, "And you are there." Unfortunately I wasn't, at least for this story, which is a doozie. I'd heard about it years ago, and I eventually met a physician who said that he'd actually witnessed it when the patient walked into his ER. To the best of my recollection, here's the story.

Contemplating the cause of his mental illness, Jack decided that his troubles were rooted in his liver. After this brilliant diagnosis, he crafted an easy fix: remove his liver. He performed the operation using only local anesthesia, numbing successive layers of tissue as he progressed through his abdomen. He eventually made it down to the liver, but found that he couldn't freeze the area well enough to make the pain bearable. So he walked into an ER and asked for help. I can't recall his exact words, but I think it was something such as, "Excuse me, I'm having some difficulty removing my liver. Can you help?"

■ I didn't know whether to laugh or to cry. I'd just pronounced a man dead who had sustained a cardiac arrest at home. His wife witnessed the arrest, but didn't immediately call 911. Instead, she got out a chrome-plated ring-shaped contraption. The outer ring held another ring which in turn held balls which were spun by the user (I may have botched the description of this gizmo, but it's something equally absurd). She placed this device over his chest, and spun the balls. Again, and again, and again. As her husband's life slowly ebbed away, she kept spinning the balls. Eventually, she called 911.

As every adult of normal intelligence knows, rapid response is vital to the success of cardiac resuscitation. Delaying a 911 call to perform voodoo rituals is tantamount to murder. This man's fate was sealed by his wife's stupidity. There is no other way to put it; no other way to dilute the noxiousness of that fact.

She seemed to sincerely believe in the utility of her act. She even provided me with a scientific explanation of how the device worked. Clearly, the device didn't work, and there was no science behind it—just superstition. This man was dead, and there was no bringing him back to life. Fearing that she might perform her ritual on someone else, I was compelled to explain to her that such a practice could not help. Furthermore, by delaying care, it would undoubtedly hurt. I recommended that she enroll in a CPR (cardiopulmonary resuscitation) course. I tried to phrase this in such a way that she would not feel guilty about what she'd done to her husband, but so she would realize this was something she should never do again. I don't know if I succeeded, but it was something which needed to be said.

■ Stacy presented to the ER complaining of lower abdominal pain. As a routine part of the medical history, I asked whether or not she was sexually active. She looked a bit embarrassed, then replied, "No, I don't have a *lot* of sex—just a couple of times per week."

■ The nurse's voice resounded with scorn. "Those are fake seizures. What a crock!" Whether Betty had ever sustained a real seizure was anyone's guess, but she had a long track record at this hospital of presenting with fake seizures. This seizure looked hokey as well, so I performed a few tests to determine whether or not the seizure was genuine. The nurse was correct; it *was* fake. After I curtly informed Betty that her charade was over, she immediately sat up and said, "OK, but before you discharge me, can I have a snack?"

■ When I was a medical student in Detroit, we had two patients in the ER at the same time, each of whom claimed to be Jesus. As is usually the case with such patients, neither of these fellows was shy about their proclamation. They would scream at every passerby, "*I am **Jesus**! You shall kneel before me!*" or something similar. After a few hours, this became quite irksome. Then one of the staff members had a nifty solution: put both men in the same room, and let them argue with each other. "I'm Jesus!" "No, you can't be Jesus, because *I'm* Jesus!" It went on for hours.

■ Now *this* could be interesting, I thought to myself. Ron and Pam were on the first night of their honeymoon, and both were registered as patients. They looked too healthy to have food poisoning, and the fact that they were holding hands led me to believe they hadn't been arguing. Pam seemed a bit sheepish, but Ron was eager to talk.

**Ron:** Hi, Doc. We're on our honeymoon, and we're having a marital problem.

**Dr. Pezzi:** Yes?

**Ron:** We're not able to consummate our marriage.

**Dr. Pezzi:** What seems to be the problem?

**Ron:** I can't get it in her.

**Dr. Pezzi:** Are you able to get an erection?

**Ron:** Heck, yeah. It was hard as a rock. I just couldn't get it in—it just didn't want to go.

**Dr. Pezzi:** (looking at Pam) Have you ever had intercourse?

**Pam:** No, I'm a virgin.

At this point in time, I thought it was most likely that she had vaginismus, which means that the muscles around the vagina were in spasm; such a contraction can make penetration difficult or impossible. Vaginismus is generally rooted in a psychological aversion to coitus. Alternatively, I thought that her hymen might be the source of the problem. I discussed these possibilities with them. As I was about to find out, Ron was a creative thinker.

**Ron:** I've got an idea, Doc.

**Dr. Pezzi:** What's that?

**Ron:** Wouldn't it help if she was unconscious?

**Dr. Pezzi:** Do you mean asleep?

**Ron:** No, *unconscious.*

**Dr. Pezzi:** Well, yes, it would probably help, but how do you propose to do that? (I was wondering if he was planning on getting her plastered with booze.)

**Ron:** Can't you put her out? You know, anesthetize her?

**Dr. Pezzi:** (shocked) *What?*

**Ron:** Yeah, anesthetize her, and I'd get it in when she's out.

**Dr. Pezzi:** I can't do that!

**Pam:** It's OK with me.

**Dr. Pezzi:** I still can't do it. It's just not proper.

**Pam:** But I'd do anything for Ron. I love him.

**Dr. Pezzi:** I'm sure that you do, but that's not the issue. The logical thing to do at this juncture is for me to examine Pam. Let's try to determine the cause of the problem before we consider any solutions, alright?

**Ron:** Yeah, that makes sense.

As I performed the pelvic examination, it didn't take me long to realize why Ron was having difficulty entering her, but I didn't want to say anything until Ron was back in the room.  A few minutes later, we were all back together.

**Dr. Pezzi:**  Pam, you've never had a period, have you?

**Pam:**  Not yet.

**Dr. Pezzi:**  Did you ever see your doctor about that?

**Pam:**  No.

**Dr. Pezzi:**  Did your Mom's obstetrician ever say anything special to her after you were born?

**Pam:**  I was delivered by old Doc Martin.  He died about ten years ago, and I don't think he ever said anything to my parents—at least, nothing they ever told me.

**Ron:**  (emphatically) Why?  What's wrong?

**Dr. Pezzi:**  (thinking, *oh boy, how do I phrase this?*)  Well, when I did the exam, Pam's external genitals looked normal, but . . .

**Ron:**  *But what?!?*

**Dr. Pezzi:**  Her vagina is not normally developed.

**Ron:**  What do you mean by that?

**Dr. Pezzi:**  She doesn't have a vagina . . .

**Ron:**  Holy shit!!!

**Pam:**  (momentarily stunned, then began crying) I don't have one?

**Dr. Pezzi:**  Not a normal vagina.  Her vulva opens into a pouch that is at most an inch deep, and there's no uterus.

**Pam:**  (still sobbing) You mean I'm not a *woman?*

**Dr. Pezzi:**  (thinking that this isn't the time for a lecture on genetics and abnormal androgen receptors)  You *are* a woman . . .

**Ron:**  Oh, thank goodness! (pause)  Then why doesn't she have a vagina?

Pam had the testicular feminization syndrome (TFS).  This results when a fetus that is *genetically* a *male* lacks a receptor for testosterone, which prevents the body from responding to the testosterone.  Since testosterone is responsible for the development of male sexual characteristics, absence of its effect blocks the appearance of the male "equipment."  Sans the testosterone effect, the body is programmed to develop more or less as a

75

female—at least externally. In fact, one of my professors said that women with TFS are often unusually attractive, and he claimed that women who are cover models for *Cosmopolitan* and similar magazines are far more likely to have TFS than a woman with average looks. Sounds like an interesting research project, if nothing else.

Internally, it's another story. Some TFS women have a short, rudimentary vagina, but the other plumbing just isn't there. Hence, they cannot conceive.

Although they were hungry for a thorough explanation, I thought it was best to obscure the fact that Pam was, at least genetically, a male. I explained how she could develop a vagina which would allow them to have intercourse, and I emphasized that she was essentially just a woman who would be permanently infertile. She would need some additional treatment, but they could otherwise lead a normal life together.

They seemed relieved. So was I.

■ I was explaining to the patient that he'd probably need surgery. He raised his eyebrows. "Surgery?"

"Yes, I think so."

"*Forget it!*" he screamed.

"Why'd you say that?" I asked.

"You want me to tell you about the last time I had surgery?"

"Sure."

"I was *awake* during the surgery. They forgot to put me to sleep. I felt everything! It was torture! I've had nightmares ever since!"

Such cases are rare, but they do occur. When people are given general anesthesia (i.e., "put to sleep"), they are basically given two types of drugs: one to paralyze the muscles during surgery, and one to relieve pain and make the person unconscious. If an inadequate dose of the latter drug is given, a patient can be awake during surgery, feeling every slice and stitch, but he can't scream or even bat his eyes. Imagine that.

■ As I walked into Kurt's room, I couldn't help but notice that he looked sheepish. I introduced myself, and asked how I could be of assistance.

**Kurt:** Uh, well . . . well, I cut myself while I was working on my car.

**Dr. Pezzi:** OK. What did you cut?

**Kurt:** Ummm . . . do I have to tell you?

**Dr. Pezzi:** I'm bound to find out sooner or later.

**Kurt:** Well, I cut my penis.

**Dr. Pezzi:** (Noticing his heavy overalls.) How did you do that?

**Kurt:** I, uh . . . well, I . . . I stuck my penis in the carburetor.

**Dr. Pezzi:** You put your penis in the *carburetor*?

**Kurt:** Yeah, while the engine was running.

**Dr. Pezzi:** (Thinking what a lonely guy he must be.) Why did you do that?

**Kurt:** Well, I was horny.

**Dr. Pezzi:** (No kidding, I thought to myself.) Weren't you concerned?

**Kurt:** No. The sperm would just burn up in the engine. It wouldn't hurt the motor.

**Dr. Pezzi:** (Wondering how much I could make by submitting this story to the *National Enquirer*, or some other noted repository of human normality.) No, when I asked if you were concerned, I was referring to the potential danger to you, not to your engine.

**Kurt:** Heck, no. My cousin has been doing it for years, and he's never been hurt.

**Dr. Pezzi:** (I mused, doesn't anyone in his family like women?) Was this the first time you tried it?

**Kurt:** No, I'd done it before with my old GMC pickup, but my cousin told me that my Ford would have more suction.

**Dr. Pezzi:** (Realizing what a disappointment that must be to Mr. Goodwrench.) You don't intend to do this again, do you?

**Kurt:** Not with that Ford.

**Dr. Pezzi:** (Ah, monogamy!) But with the GMC?

**Kurt:** I don't know. Maybe.

**Dr. Pezzi:** (Deciding that I have to formally warn him, so as to limit my liability for any subsequent injuries to his penis caused by carburetor copulation.) From a medical standpoint, what you've been doing is extremely dangerous. Aside from the risk of injury to your penis, you could be injured in many other ways, or even killed.

**Kurt:** Yeah, I know that, but it feels so good.

**Dr. Pezzi:** It does? That's difficult to believe.

**Kurt:** Yes, it does. Don't knock it until you've tried it.

Meanwhile, back on planet Earth . . . After finishing with Kurt, I walked over to the nursing station. Marci, the clerk, told me that one of the local television stations had called, wondering if we had any interesting cases they could do a story on. I doubted that this would fit in well on the six o'clock news, and I doubted that Kurt would be eager to publicize his penile proclivities. "No, Marci, just the usual stuff. Nothing newsworthy."

■ I don't know where this fellow had come from, but I'm sure it wasn't a Mensa meeting. Barry walked out of a building and over to a Pontiac Fiero (back in the days when that was *the* car to have) without first checking to see who was around. How Barry failed to notice the police cruiser parked behind the Fiero is beyond me. Naturally, Barry drew their attention when he smashed the Fiero's side window to gain access to the car. Barry started the car and took off, and so did the police.

While Fieros may have looked sporty, they weren't particularly fast cars. Eventually, Barry realized that he would not be able to outrun the police, so he decided to jump out of the vehicle while it was still moving . . . at 85 m.p.h., according to the police. That was his second major mistake of the day. His third major mistake occurred when he failed to pick a soft spot for his landing; when Barry jumped from the vehicle, he flew smack dab into a telephone pole. Now comatose, he was brought into the ER so that we could save him. I thought it was futile to even try.

# *Solved & Unsolved Mysteries*

■ An unconscious 30-year-old man was brought to the ER by ambulance. His girlfriend found him lying naked on the floor of his bathroom, and called 911. In the ER, he was found to have a large lump on the top of his head and, strangely, several scratches on his scrotum. The lump was not much of an enigma, and probably explained why he was knocked out, but the source of the scratches remained a mystery until he woke up and provided us with the following explanation. He said he had been cleaning his bathtub while naked, kneeling on the floor beside the tub. His cat, apparently transfixed by the rhythmic swaying of his scrotum, lunged forward, sinking its claws into this pendulous target. This caused the man to rocket upward, striking his head on the top frame of the shower door. Mystery solved.

■ A 40-ish man had been found unconscious in his car, which was in the median of the freeway. There had been no accident or other trauma, no heart attack, no booze, and no drugs. In short, there was no explanation.

He was brought to the ER for evaluation, and I did everything I could think of to evaluate him: dozens of blood and urine tests, an EKG and heart monitoring, a CAT scan and various x-rays, and a thorough examination. Still, he remained comatose, and we didn't know why. From his clothes, address, and membership in various ritzy clubs, we knew he had money. His wallet gave us such trivial details, but nothing to help us solve the puzzle: no medical information cards, and no doctor or relative to contact in case of emergency. Every path we followed came to a dead end, so he was admitted to the Intensive Care Unit, still comatose.

The next day, he suddenly woke up and said, "What the heck am I doing here?" He put his clothes on and left. The cause for his coma was never determined.

■ For reasons that are not clear to me, women who are strippers (or "professional dancers," as they prefer to call themselves) seem compelled to inform me of their occupation within the first ten seconds of my meeting them in the ER. Thrusting out their right hand (and sometimes other parts of their anatomy), their introductions have an eerie similarity, as if this skill was taught to them in stripping school. "Hi! I'm Veronica! I'm a professional dancer . . ." End of the intro, and long pause. Perhaps they're waiting for me to say something, but I'm not bright enough to figure out what it is they're looking for. Adulation? Sorrow? A request for an autograph, maybe? I dunno.

It's not that I dislike strippers. If anything, their candid bluntness is a pleasing departure from the all-too-frequent repartee of bullshit which often blocks effective communication between the patient and the ER doctor. Most strippers know that they're willingly debasing themselves by engaging in humiliating work, but they are at a loss to find a more respectable job that pays equally well. In that respect, they're like ER doctors.

When I read the triage note[12] on Diane, I speculated, "I bet it's LGV." A nurse who was standing beside me at the nursing station inquired, "What's LGV?"[13]

"*This* is LGV," I immediately recognized as I entered the patient's cubicle. Diane didn't bother to don the gown, much to my eternal gratitude. She was obviously comfortable being naked—an occupational benefit, perhaps. While the physiques of most strippers often left me wondering why men would pay to see them, Diane's beauty left me stunned. But it's not polite to stare, so I went right on with the questioning. The mystery wasn't *what* she had, but *how* she'd acquired it. She said that she wasn't having sex. Ordinarily, since LGV is a sexually transmitted disease (STD), I'd question her veracity. Furthermore, I'd guessed that she must have had dozens of men chasing after her. The fact that she wasn't having sex may seem implausible, but I believed her. By denying it, what would she be trying to protect—her reputation? Obviously, she was quite comfortable with herself and her chosen occupation. Fibbing about her sexual life seemed to be a non sequitur.

A few minutes into the questioning, she said that she and several other strippers had shared a G-string last month. One person took it off, and another immediately put it on. Gee whiz, and I'd been warned to never share a toothbrush or comb with anyone (I gleaned these personal hygiene tips from reading my Dad's World War II Army manuals when I was in

---

[12]    This is the note written by the triage nurse, who is generally the first professional you encounter after walking into the ER. The note summarizes your complaints, and sometimes includes relevant positive and negative responses elicited by the nurse in the pursuit of their primary job: to figure out which patients need to be seen immediately, and which can wait. In general, nurses do an excellent job in separating the wheat from the chaff.

[13]    LGV (lymphogranuloma venereum) is a sexually transmitted disease caused by a certain germ (*Chlamydia trachomatis*), which results in enlargement of the inguinal lymph nodes. Occasionally, the tissue between the lymph node and the skin is eroded, with the subsequent discharge of pus. A pretty site, it's not.

third grade). Uh, sharing a G-string . . . *without washing?* OK, so she's not a rocket scientist.

Combine a G-string, soaked with the secretions of prior users, with the rubbing and tugging upon it which seems to be a necessary aspect of such titillation, and what do you get? An efficient means of spreading STDs without the need for intercourse. I'd solved the mystery of how she had acquired the infection, but I was still mystified by her lack of common sense. Or, maybe she never read her Dad's Army manuals?

■ Steve complained of a headache. Routine questioning failed to uncover any apparent reason for the headache in this 12-year-old patient, so I began my examination. It didn't take long to hit pay dirt. As I was palpating his scalp, I noticed something projecting out of it. Brushing his hair aside, I immediately recognized what it was.

**Dr. Pezzi:** How long have you had this bullet in your head, Steve?

**Steve:** What bullet?

**Dr. Pezzi:** This bullet that's half-embedded in your skull.

**Steve:** I don't have a bullet in my head.

**Dr. Pezzi:** Yes you do. It's right here.

**Steve:** Are you sure?

**Dr. Pezzi:** Yes, I'm sure. How did this happen?

**Steve:** I don't know.

**Dr. Pezzi:** You don't remember being shot?

**Steve:** Nope. I've never been shot.

I found it rather difficult to believe that a person could be shot and not notice it. Even if the gun with which he was shot had a silencer, or the gun was a considerable distance from him (which would explain why the bullet had not fully penetrated his skull), it would not be easy to miss the recognition of pain as the bullet tore through the scalp and the outer layer of the skull. Imagine someone hammering a quarter-inch diameter nail into your head; think you'd notice it?

# *Your tax dollars, hard at work*

While most of the stories in this section are not as funny or as purely entertaining as the stories in other sections of this book, I think that it is eminently worthwhile to read this material. To begin with, some of the stories *are* funny. In fact, a couple of my all-time favorite stories are in this section. Secondly, some of these stories are a prerequisite to fully appreciating the humor in subsequent sections. Finally, it is inconceivable to me that this material would not be of interest to all responsible citizens. While I have no qualms about providing necessary medical care, I am abhorred by the colossal amount of money that is being wasted by a variety of scams, schemes, and fraudulent practices. Virtually all of my colleagues (and certainly all hospital administrators) are all too happy to simply pocket the money and keep quiet, which I think is an ethical abomination. There's a tacit understanding in the healthcare industry that such waste is to be condoned, simply because there is money to be made. On the pretense of being fine, upstanding citizens, the entrenched powers keep mum, and they keep pocketing your money.

■ Patients drive the following cars to the ER: a Corvette, a brand-new Cadillac, an expensive van, and a Jeep Grand Cherokee. *Question:* Besides being expensive, what's the other striking similarity? *Answer:* They're all driven by people on Medicaid. There is a good chance that you don't have a Cadillac, but I guarantee you that you're supporting people who drive Cadillacs. Fair? You may not have air conditioning, but your tax dollars are paying for air conditioners (and the money that it costs to run them) so that people on welfare are more comfortable *than you*. Fair? Most of the welfare recipients I've met receive cable TV. Since when is the reception of 60 channels a necessity of life? They should spend their time reading the want ads and looking for a job, not watching reruns of *The Brady Bunch!*

A Medicaid recipient visited the ER because she believed that she had contracted food poisoning from a steak she had eaten earlier in the day at a local restaurant. Her husband and eight kids, all of whom were also on Medicaid, shared in the same feast. I'll bet that many of the taxpayers who purchased this meal sat at home that night, eating Hamburger Helper®, so these ten Medicaid recipients could eat steak! Clearly, if they're eating steak, they're being "paid" too much. Eating *steak* at a *restaurant* is a luxury, not a necessity of life. When I was younger, there were times I was so poor that I envied people "wealthy enough" to eat at McDonald's®! In fact, that was one of my reasons for going into medicine. A doctor, I figured, could eat at McDonald's® whenever he wished. Well, my culinary ideals have since changed, but I never asked anyone to buy me a meal, even when my stomach was growling in hunger. I knew that some day I'd *earn* the money that would allow me to eat well. Other people, obviously, are not so disciplined. They are content to elect politicians who will figuratively hold you at gunpoint to make you pay enough taxes so they can afford luxuries like steak, while you're choking on peanut butter! When will this madness end?

There's more. A 32-year-old man and his girlfriend came into the ER last winter, both saying that they strained their backs while snowmobiling. This might not seem unusual, except that they're both on Medicaid. If a person is so destitute as to "deserve" Medicaid, how can they afford a snowmobile, snowmobile suits and helmets, upkeep of the snowmobile, and money for gas, oil, insurance, and registration fees? Snowmobiling is an expensive hobby—it's a *luxury*, not a necessity. Furthermore, the man is on permanent Social Security disability for a supposed back injury! If his back is so bad that he can't work, what is he doing on a snowmobile? Scam, *scam, scam!* Your tax dollars, hard at work. I've seen so many Medicaid cards pulled from $400 designer purses that I've even considered becoming a politician, in the hope of terminating such profligate waste. You're working your butt off to pay taxes so that people on public assistance can afford luxuries that you cannot afford; is this fair?

■ While speaking with a 28-year-old man who had come to the ER for a minor problem, I noticed on the chart, in the employment box, that he was "disabled." Curiosity got the best of me, and I asked this man—who had no obvious impairments—how he was disabled. "My doctor says I can't ever work, 'cause if I do, the noise might damage my hearing." That's funny, I thought, since noise can damage *anyone's* hearing. Why don't we all just retire and sponge off the government? Furthermore, not all jobs involve exposure to loud noise. Why not just get a quiet job? This being obvious, I'm debating which is more execrable: the contemptible absence of ambition in this person, or the criminally negligent declaration of "disability" from the doctor. What a scam. The doctor profits either by taking a cut of the welfare loot, or by "treating" such a patient for an interminable series of imaginary problems. Ah, the great American pastime . . . the fleecing of America.

■ A long, long time ago, in a land unfortunately not far enough away, I had the distinct displeasure of meeting a family so bizarre that it's difficult to convey in words just how strange these people were—but I'll try, anyway. Dad and Mom brought in their teenage daughters, both odd, but only one of whom was registered as a patient. Upset about the lack of attention given to her earlier in the day by her boyfriend, the patient decided that life was no longer worth living, so she took an "overdose" of sleeping pills. Actually, the amount that she took wouldn't faze a chipmunk, but I sensed the presence of enough psychopathology in this person to warrant investigation. After initiating the usual CYA medical evaluation, the taxpayers were out of another $1000—the entire family was on welfare . . . surprised?—and nothing unusual turned up. Gotta placate the lawyers, though.

Trying to ignore the incorrigibility of this patient's neuroses, which have proven refractory to prior counseling, I called in a psychologist under the guise of evaluating this patient, but what I really wanted was a psychological dissection of the family unit, which was manifestly unbalanced. With the patient's last overdose, the patient informed her parents that she refused to go to the emergency room, to which the parents said, "OK." So much for putting their feet down and asserting parental authority.

Psychological evaluations take time, especially when the mining turns up gold, so the patient was in the ER for several hours. Early on, it became apparent that the parents wanted to take their depressed daughter back home, into the nurturing milieu which imparted her amazingly adaptive behavioral patterns. I nixed that idea, lacking confidence in the ability of pathology to cure pathology. To their credit, the parents seemed to appreciate that the aberrant dynamics of their family were not amenable to Band-Aid® therapy, so they agreed to postpone the taxi ride home with their daughter in tow.

Under the mistaken belief that all was well in Whoville, I was chilling out at the nursing station, when what to my wondering ears should appear, but the sound of a chair, crashing quite near. Near the epicenter of this earthquake, I found the Dad, beating a chair into submission. That accomplished, he stormed out of the emergency room, crash, boom, banging all the way. Apparently content with his victory, he returned a few minutes later, smiling, peaceful, and smugly basking in the appreciation of his deed. Thinking that it might be a good idea to see what the **H** was going on, I moseyed on over to the patient's room, finding the entire family behaving as if they had just returned from a rewarding PTA meeting. Pleased with the restoration of apparent normalcy, but at a loss to explain the emotional channel surfing, I put my trepidation level up a notch, to Defcon 4.

A succession of similarly inexplicable outbursts later, I decided that the critical mass of collective insanity was nearing the point of mushrooming out of control, so I checked out of the Marcus Welby mode and pleasantly but firmly laid out the game plan. No, patient, you're not going to pull out your IV. No, patient, you're not going to get dressed and walk out of the ER. I expected the usual resistant flak from the patient, but I was surprised when the Mom began echoing the defiance of the patient, regressively chiming in, "You can't make her stay! You can't make her stay!" Egging her on, she began encouraging her daughter to pull out the IV, put her street clothes on, and leave. Enough is enough. Defcon 3. Mom, if you want to stay, you can't continue escalating the Cold War. Mom doesn't listen. Defcon 2, the bombers are on their way. Our obviously quaint tourist town is blessed by the presence of the state, county, and city police, each of whom sent one or more ambassadors of goodwill. Unbeknownst to me at the time, the patient's sister had been convicted of assaulting the daughter of one of the police officers who had responded to the ER. Oh, no, bad blood. Defcon 1. I witnessed the evaporation of whatever internal restraints remained in this family, who then gave free reign to their limbic impulses. Threats melted into action, and flailing arms met handcuffs. Dad, Mom, and sister soon discovered that hospital visitors are not protected by Diplomatic Immunity, so their egress from the hospital was facilitated by the police. Oh, Mom feigned passing out as she's leaving, but she didn't receive my vote for an Academy Award. I checked her out, and she left. Before the curtain fell on her performance for the night, though, I asked the Mom why she put up such a vicious fight with the police. "Did you see the *panties* on my daughter? Did you see her *legs*?" Sensing that it was most prudent to view such inquiries as rhetorical questions, I remained silent. Anxious to provide me with the nexus which might pardon the behavior of her family, the Mom continued her exegesis. "If any man saw her legs or her sexy panties, he wouldn't be able to control himself!"

As if she sensed the necessity of providing a further explanation to root such paranoia with reality, she told me that she feared the remaining police officers would, sans Mom, rape her daughter. To paraphrase the eloquence of General Anthony McAuliffe at the Battle of the Bulge, nuts. Hmmm, let's see, the officers are going to throw away their marriages, their morality, their careers, spend the rest of their lives in state prison, and risk the acquisition of an assortment of venereal diseases (the patient admitted to a history of prostitution), all for the pleasure of mating with an unbalanced teenager of questionable pulchritude? This stretched the limits of credibility just a tad, and such logic failed to impress me.

I looked over at the patient, and she was seething. Somewhere along the way, she had managed to rearrange some of the internal anatomy of one of our ER staff members, Kim, who sustained a fracture when Kim discovered that the patient's sister was not kidding when she was gloating about how hard her sister, the patient, could kick. Call me old-fashioned, but I could not concur with these folks that vicious kicking should be a point of family pride. But it was for them, nonetheless. The patient was bristling with indignation that the fractured staff member would have the temerity to press charges, no doubt convinced that a person of her caliber should not be affronted with the need to be held accountable for her actions.

Such gall! Ah, the wacky world of welfare. Feed me, clothe me, care for me, and meekly lay down as I walk all over you. Doesn't it give you a warm feeling when you realize that the existence of such lunacy is being perpetuated by your tax dollars?

■ Years ago, phrenologists attempted to discover correlations between the size and protuberances of a person's skull and their character and mental capacity. While phrenology has been discredited, it is clear that certain somatic attributes *are* associated with intellectual, behavioral, and economic traits. Let's not muddy the waters with an attempt, à la the temporal dilemma in the chicken or the egg conundrum, to clarify the genesis of the variables. Instead, let's consider the correlations themselves, unfettered from any extraneous considerations. Correlation #1: the sloth/mega-tummy association. People who have somehow failed to receive the genetic honing that's accrued over the past 100,000 years seem more likely to possess certain undesirable intellectual and behavioral features that are correlated with the presence of a massive lower belly ("tummy"). Now, I can understand how women can acquire somewhat of a tummy after they've been pregnant, but I'm not referring to your run-of-the-mill paunch—I'm talking about a gravity-defying horizontal projection of adipose tissue of bewildering magnitude. Having worked for years in emergency rooms, I've seen more than my share of obesity, but when I meet a profane, unkempt, unemployed, unisyllabic, edentulous Medicaid recipient, that person has a much greater-than-average chance of possessing a blimp-like lower abdomen that never fails to leave my eyes, jaded as they are to the sight of blubber, stupefied in disbelief. Logically, one might assume that such a person, theoretically lacking the ability to purchase—and chew—a steak, would be more apt to manifest signs of starvation. Incidentally, this enigma is not gender-specific; I've seen hundreds of males whose lower abdominal size suggested Goodyear® ancestry.

Correlation #2: the welfare/inbred*-look and/or moronic* lineage association[14] (*: these terms are intended literally, not pejoratively). A cousin of the above, pun intended. Most jokes have some basis in reality, and the jokes about inbreeding are no exception, except they're no laughing matter. Marry your cousin, and Jimmy the Greek will not go broke betting that your offspring will not be cheerleaders in college. The pleasant city in which I live and work is, unfortunately, surrounded by a number of towns in which inbreeding seems to be the predominant means of reproduction. When the denizens of those areas come to the ER, their unique phenotypic aberrations signal that yet another resident of the inbred belt has arrived, clutching their Medicaid card as they mindlessly and shamelessly pillage the bank accounts of working Americans, never evincing the slightest bit of compunction for their unrequited greed. Functionally almost anencephalic[15], it is perhaps not too surprising that their visits to the ER are typically for less-than-legitimate reasons.

A case in point. A 30-year-old man came to the ER with a kidney stone; so far, a legitimate ER visit . . . but just wait. Upon evaluation, the stone was found to be small, and his pain was easily controlled with analgesics (pain-relieving medicine). He was discharged with pain pills that he was instructed to take if his pain recurred. If his pain continued after taking the pills, he was told to return to the ER. Simple? Not for him. He returned later in the day, saying that his pain had recurred. I asked him if he had taken one of the pain pills, and he said, "No." He was given one of the pain pills, and felt fine. I then asked him why he didn't take the analgesic, and he responded, "I didn't know that you wanted me to *take them*." What did he think, that I wanted him to *stare* at the pills in the bottle? I, once again, explained what he should do at home if his pain recurred. This thought, apparently reverberating through the vacuum in his skull, didn't sink in. He began complaining about the need to drive back to the ER if his pain recurred after the current medicine had worn off. Again, I explained that this would be an indication for taking another pain pill, and the patient seemed astonished, as if I'd been explaining the workings of a

---

[14]    To those who doubt the veracity of such a correlation, I offer the following challenge: put your money where your mouth is. I am not asseverating that such a correlation is good or bad, only that it exists, and that I can predict, at a rate which is statistically significant, such correlations by phenotypic extrapolation. I bet $1,000,000.00; any takers?

[15]    No brain.

perpetual motion machine. No Nobel Prize for him. Stunned at his inability to grasp such a basic concept, I began wondering how he had the sense to open a cupboard and retrieve food when he was hungry.

Since beauty is in the eye of the beholder, I will not elaborate upon the physical aberrations that are associated with inbreeding. Suffice it to say that, even in the absence of major defects, inbreeding produces people who have a characteristic look. Enamored as I am with intelligence, and in realization of the fact that some of the greatest minds in history have been housed in defective bodies, I view the physical defects as a minor problem to society as a whole. While such defects may be distressing to the individual (if they have enough intelligence to appreciate them), their societal impact is negligible. Unfortunately, the same cannot be said about the associated mental aberrations, which are the greatest nemesis to civilization since the plague. As you will soon realize, I'm *not* kidding about this matter.

The survival of any species, including man, is predicated upon the fact that individuals with the most adaptive traits are the most likely to survive and eventually reproduce. Animals with physical or mental defects are not apt to survive to reproductive age, and hence have little chance of passing their genes to subsequent generations. Until recently, the same was also true of humans. The legislated coddling of the incompetent via welfare in this century has permitted the survival and reproduction of individuals that, if they were left to make it on their own, otherwise simply could not survive. If such people reproduced at a rate proportional to their existing percentage of the population, this would not be much of a problem. However, they currently have a disproportionately high rate of reproduction. Stated another way, there is an inverse correlation of reproduction with intelligence. I've never seen an intelligent 20-year-old mother with six children, but I've seen countless feeble-minded mothers of that age waddle into the ER with their entire family, seeking treatment for one and all. "Bobby got bit by a moskeeter [mosquito]. Sally got some bugs in her hair, and Jimmy done got some warts on his fingers. Billy, he been a coughin', and Sam there been sneezin'. Katie been havin' the runs, and I be havin' a discharge, ya know, down there, and I thinks maybe I be pregnant." If the artificially-enabled reproductive success of people of that ilk continues for a few thousand years, the average intelligence of mankind will plummet. Humans are not the largest, fastest, or strongest species on Earth; our survival is dependent upon our one supreme attribute: brainpower. Dilute that, and we're goners. As it is, mankind is never more than one mutation away from extinction. A single nondescript germ, a few continents away from your condo in New York, could mutate into a virulent killing machine that wipes out the entire human race in short order. You've heard of AIDS, you've heard of Ebola, but you haven't heard the last of the germs. Sooner or later, some bug will arise that makes AIDS look like the common cold. It's a good guess that the solution to such a problem will not spring from the mind of a moron. If the average human intelligence is halved, and this is possible, virtually *everyone* will be a moron. Notwithstanding our limited technological success in the present, such people of the future would be unable to reap the benefits of today's technology because they would be too stupid to read and understand what we have already accomplished. If a modern-day welfare recipient is challenged by the concept of swallowing a pill, is it reasonable to expect that his progeny, with half his intelligence a few thousand years hence, will devise a drug to combat the new plague?

I realize many liberals are abhorred by any discussion of genetics which suggests that humans are not immune to intellectual decrement when mentally inferior individuals are reproducing at a disproportionately high rate. However, ignoring this problem, in the manner of the ostrich fable, will not make it go away. The perpetuation and furtherance of idiocy, unless checked, will mean the extinction of mankind.

■ Speaking of idiocy, I am reminded of the following story. A 26-year-old man came into the ER, complaining of—*drum roll, please*—belly button lint. Where's Mr. Ripley when you need him, eh? Upon inspection, there was no infection or other problems, just plain ol' belly button lint. You really have to wonder about such a fellow, sitting at home, realizing, "Hmmm . . . I've got lint in my belly button. I'd better go to the emergency room." Sorry, buddy, your application for membership in Mensa has been rejected. His rich and rewarding life was made possible by—what else?—welfare.

■ When I began working in the ER years ago, I had no preconceived notions about people on welfare. I'd once been dirt poor, and I didn't think there was any difference between welfare recipients and me, except for a bit of pride. Boy, was I wrong! Now, I'm not going to make an overgeneralization and claim that all people who receive public assistance are "different," but I've seen enough of them who are to make me, reluctantly, a believer in stereotypes. Deep down, I don't like to stereotype people. Always the eternal optimist, I'm forever looking to disprove my conceptions about welfare folks. Trouble is, they're continually reinforcing my stereotype—not decimating it.

The clean-slate opinion with which I began the practice of medicine was rapidly molded by exposure to "welfarites." In addition to their other traits, I've often found them to be obnoxiously demanding. When I was younger, my bias was against rich people who, I assumed, would snootily make all sorts of demands. This latter prejudice dissipated when I found that it was baseless. On the other hand, when someone is stomping his foot, demanding this or that, that person is almost invariably a welfarite. This strikes me as odd. Whatever happened to the idea that "beggars can't be choosers"? Whatever happened to gratitude? Oh, forget gratitude—I'd be happy if they would just stop their uncouth behavior.

Maxine fit the stereotype. I'd guess that she was about 38, but her gaunt, edentulous face made her appear much older. When I walked into the room, I noticed an *I-want-to-kill-you* look on her face. I smiled, hoping for a reflexive social de-escalation of her rage. No luck. Apart from her frightening countenance, I was struck by the overwhelming stench of cigarettes. She didn't just reek of smoke, she smelled as if she had been soaking in a vat of nicotine and tar for the past few decades. Maxine had brought her infant to the ER, saying that the baby had a cold for the past two weeks. She hadn't made an appointment with the pediatrician, but, inexplicably, she decided all of a sudden that the child needed to be brought to the ER. What possessed her to arrive at that conclusion, I do not know. The baby was happy, smiling, active, and playful. When I would smile at him, he would look absolutely joyous, and smile back. The examination was utterly unremarkable. From the history, it seemed that the child had indeed *had* a cold, but he was obviously now over it.

I explained to Maxine that she could minimize the chance of future illness in her baby by not smoking inside her home. This, she haughtily told me as if I were a second-grade scientific neophyte, had nothing to do with the cold. Lisping, she said that she burned a candle whenever she smoked. The flame of the candle, she claimed, "sucked up all of the smoke in the house." Such erudition! Such a breakthrough! Not only will this eliminate the health risks of secondhand smoke, it's a surefire means of preventing deaths due to smoke inhalation in building fires. Yup, we'll just all keep a candle burning. If there is any smoke, the candle flame will just "suck it up." Problem solved! I felt sorry for the child. With a mother that vacuous, he was bound to be victimized by a string of other wacky ideas.

Having done precious little to impress me with her intelligence, Maxine wasted no time in pronouncing that I was wrong about her child. She implored, "Can't you see how sick my baby is?" Oh, I get it—the baby is ill, and he's just *pretending* to be healthy and happy. Clever little thing, he's just trying to spoof me! Maxine then insisted that she receive a second opinion. "Is there another doctor working—I want someone else to check my baby!" I explained that there was not another doctor working in the ER. Somehow, this hospital trusted me to take care of patients on my own, even patients who were gravely ill or injured. Medically, this was not a challenging case. "Well then," she continued, "I want my own doctor in here, and I want him in here NOW!"

I called the child's doctor, who graciously came to the ER. He checked the patient thoroughly, and agreed with my prior conclusions. I wasn't looking for vindication, but I was happy that the groundless consternation of the mother was assuaged. Her fears may have been put to rest, but her anger was still in full force. On her way home, she stopped at a pay phone and called the ER. The ER registration clerk fielded the call.

**Maxine:** I'm just calling to say how rude you, the nurse, and the doctor were!

**Clerk:** I . . . (The clerk never had a chance to defend herself, but I will. This particular clerk is more pleasant than an average game show host. Rude, she's not.)

**Maxine:** That nurse asked me to have a seat while she took care of that old fart with chest pains! I got there at the same time, and I *don't* like to wait! She should have taken me in first! I've got better things to do with my time! (Like what—cash welfare checks and waste the taxpayer's money on inane ER visits?)

I was puzzled by her proclamations of rudeness. Sensing the chip on her shoulder, I went out of my way to be pleasant. *She* was the one who was rude, as she petulantly belittled the "old fart" with chest pain, self-centeredly insisting that she go first. We acceded to all of her insolent demands, and then she had the audacity to call the hospital to bitch us out? *What a jerk!* Incidentally, I've noticed that welfarites are more likely to be the "victims" of physical assaults. I'm sure their abrasive behavior is not limited to hospitals, which often results in their being pummeled by those whom they exasperate.

One day prior to Maxine's ER visit/temper tantrum, I had another welfarite come in by ambulance after someone hit him on the head. He was in a neck brace and on a backboard, so he couldn't see me as I began to approach him. He introduced himself by threatening, "If you're a n____ (you know, the famous "N-word" in the O.J. trial), I'm gonna beat your ass!" Given that I had only said, "Hi, I'm Dr. Pezzi," this response seemed a tad strong. Where are these welfarites getting their manners from? Oh, I almost forgot.  This character also demanded that I call his doctor "at once."  What is this, genetic?

■ An 18-year-old high school senior was brought to the ER at 2 a.m. by his Mom, seeking evaluation of a "lump" that he had for the past year beneath one of his nipples.  He had unilateral gynecomastia (a typically benign one-sided enlargement of breast tissue), which is not uncommon during puberty.  He had already been evaluated by a physician and a surgeon, who told him not to worry about it.

What possessed this Medicaid family to pop into the ER in the middle of the night?  The problem hadn't changed, but he did request an excuse from school for the next day.  The patient looked to be in as much distress as if he had just been told that he got a date with Christie Brinkley, so I said no.  The nurse who was working with me was more direct, saying something that I felt but didn't have the guts to say, "You want a school excuse for *this*?  School is good for you—it keeps you off welfare!"

The ability to pop into an ER any time of the day or night, for any such "problem," is a luxury, not a necessity.  If people who are able to work were forced to compensate society for the expenses incurred as a result of their medical care, it would not be necessary to arbitrarily decide which care is necessary and which is superfluous.  Have a cut?  Have a breast lump that has already been evaluated . . . *twice*?  Got some belly button lint?  Hey, no problem, just come to the ER.  Can't pay the bill?  Hey, no problem, just put down your Nintendo® game, and for the next month mow the lawn of the widowed octogenarian on the corner, or shovel the snow off the driveway of the World War II veteran who had his arms blown off by a Nazi artillery shell.  Don't want to give anything back to the society that's helping you?  Say you won't lift a finger to help those older folks?  Hey, no problem, we'll just cut off your free medical care, your welfare check, your subsidized housing, your supplemental "disability—*I can't ever work 'cause noise might damage my hearing*" scam-income check, your food stamps, and when the batteries in your Nintendo® are drained, that's it . . . no more Pac-Man®, no more belly button lint evaluations, no more unearned freebies of any sort.  In short order, people who are accustomed to taking from society, without giving anything back, would learn the most fundamental rule in civilization—that of give and take.

■ If you want to put ER personnel into a huff, call them and say that you're thinking about coming in, but you want to see if it's busy, or you want to make an appointment (get real!), or you want to see what doctor is working.  Oh, I see . . . you're having chest pain that you think might be a heart attack.  If Dr. Jones is working, you'll rush right in; if Dr. Smith is working, you will just stay at home and ride this one out. I hope your wife passed her CPR course! Realistically, you either need emergency care, or you don't. If you find it necessary to call the ER to see if they are busy, fearing that a couple of hours in the waiting room will upset your plans for the evening, there is a good chance you don't need to be in the ER. Or, maybe, Susan Demming, the *incredibly* beautiful and talented ice skater, stopped by for a drink . . .

■ Another way of incurring the wrath of the ER staff is by attempting to disavow a reasonable level of self-responsibility. Decent people rarely try to dump their problems on the ER, but for the dregs in society, such antics are routine. For example:

> • A man in his twenties had fallen off a roof and injured his wrist. It was obviously sprained, and I suspected he might have an occult fracture. The x-rays were normal, but it is not uncommon for the initial x-rays to appear normal in certain types of wrist fractures. In such cases, it is common practice to splint the wrist as if it were fractured, and refer the patient for a follow-up examination. After I explained these points to the patient and his wife, she exclaimed, "I want you to put a cast on him, *not* a splint!" Even if this were definitely fractured, I explained, we would immobilize the area with a splint, and refer the patient to an orthopedic surgeon for casting (this is what ER doctors are taught to do in their training). "Oh, no," the wife insisted, "he's got to have a cast." Curious as to why he's "got to" have a cast, I asked for an explanation. "If you just give him a splint, he'll pull it off before we get home." If a dog pulls off a splint, I can understand that. If a two-year-old child pulls off his splint, I can understand that, too. But this is a 26-year-old man who is, presumably, an adult. For heaven's sake, exercise a smidgen of self control! "Oh, no, he will pull it right off. You'd better cast him." Feeling a sudden swell of contempt building inside, I'm sure that my countenance revealed my disgust. After more discussion, the patient agreed to leave the splint on. This nonproductive 5-minute foray into the realm of juvenile eccentricity occurred during one of the busiest days in the ER. I've noticed that on such days, a disproportionate number of odd people tend to flock to the ER.

> • "I ain't got no money to get these pills, and I ain't got nowhere to stay," lamented the unkempt middle-aged male who reeked so strongly of tobacco and cheap booze that the room in which he was standing was virtually uninhabitable. Having diligently avoided

anything that might be construed as work throughout his 40 years of life, his only apparent redeeming worth to society was that his profligate consumption of alcohol and cigarettes helped to keep liquor and tobacco companies in business. Given that he was able to beg, "borrow," and steal enough money every year to indulge in such vices and his penchant for prostitutes, I hadn't the slightest shred of sympathy for this dirtbag. Health care personnel should not be expected to fulfill the role of a parent, rich aunt, godparent, or welfare caseworker. On occasion, I have given my own money and medical goods and services to poor people that I felt were decent, deserving folks, but I don't believe in rewarding professional bums. Not everyone agrees with me, though. Years ago, I worked with a physician who would give a few dollars to a perpetually inebriated ER frequent-flyer, whenever this guy came to the ER. The money was intended to buy the boozer a meal, but alcoholics often have a warped idea of the four basic food groups, believing them to be wine, beer, liquor, and mixers. Having received his booty, the bum would announce that the medical problem which prompted his ER visit was miraculously cured, and he'd walk out of the ER with a smile on his unshaven face. Some people might view this physician's BEEFER (*B*ribe to *E*xpedite *E*gress *F*rom the *ER*) as an innocuous act, but I think otherwise. Since the boozer was rewarded for his fraudulent ER visits, he made the ER a regular inclusion in his busy schedule. Each flimflamming visit cost the American taxpayers a few hundred dollars. What a scam!

• A 20-something-year-old man presented to the ER, complaining of depression. Two hours ago, he had been at a bar, drinking with his buddies, ogling the ladies. All was well until he asked a woman to dance with him, and she turned him down. Most men would accept such a minor setback with equanimity, but this rejection threw this fellow into a vortex of despair. Did he get drunk? No. Did he ask someone else to dance? No. Did he seek solace from his friends? No. Did he scan the personal want ads? No. Did he head for the gym to work off his tension? No. Did he peruse his little black book, searching for someone more receptive? No. Instead, he came to the ER, expecting me to provide him with a solution to his libidinous desires. This pathetically execrable excuse for a man was blasted with both barrels of stinging, yet apropos advice. First, I explained that to come to the ER for such a problem was, basically, idiotic. Consoling the lovelorn was never something I considered to be within the province of emergency medicine. This character

**94**

was—*surprise!*—on welfare, and the bill for this "emergency" was footed by me, you, and other U.S. taxpayers. Second, even though I was horrified by the thought of anything that might increase the reproductive success of such a person, I decided to give him some practical advice. I nixed his suggestion that a psychiatrist might be able to help him get a date, explaining that shrinks are not magicians. Noting that he had *never* worked a day in his life, I said that women generally prefer employed men. He seemed to be mystified by this concept, retorting that he *did* have an income: the government sent him a check every month! How impressive! A job, I explained, generally supplies a valuable sense of self-worth, in addition to providing *respectable* income. Since there was no reason why this fellow couldn't work, I felt that his welfare money was morally tainted and incapable of imparting self-esteem. He felt that money is money, no matter where—or from whom—it comes from. What a loser! On to my next patient . . .

■ A nurse at a local nursing home called 911 to report that a 97-year-old resident had no pulse and wasn't breathing. The paramedics rushed over and began CPR (cardiopulmonary resuscitation). The nurse panicked and began pulling them off, shouting, *"No, no, don't do CPR!"*

Stunned, the paramedics responded, "She's not breathing. She has no pulse."

The nurse said, *"Look at these papers! See, it says that she doesn't want CPR—she doesn't want to be coded!"* This puzzled the paramedics, since the only logical reason for calling them about such a patient was to attempt resuscitation. The nurse continued, *"The family just wants her brought to the emergency room."* This also puzzled the paramedics and, once her corpse was delivered to the ER, it was no less perplexing to me. Why bring a dead person, who wants to be dead, to an ER? Let's see . . . the ambulance ride is a good $600; I have no idea what hospitals charge for their emergency doctors to officiate at rituals devoid of medical care, but I bet it's $300 or more. Give or take a hundred bucks or so, the cost of having the ER call the funeral home was $1000. Isn't this crazy? If this family was responsible for paying their own medical bills, do you think they would be so capricious in demanding that Grandma be brought to the ER for a nonexistent reason?

The next day, I had the pleasure of meeting the son of the "patient" I'd had the previous night. He presented to the ER—*via ambulance*—at 3 a.m., complaining of swollen ankles. I asked him how long he had the problem. "Eight months." Might he have seen the need to see his doctor sometime in the past few months, so that this questionable emergency visit could have been averted?  No, that would be too logical.

■ Ambulance personnel often cover patients they're transporting with a blanket to keep them warm.  As the next patient rolled into the ER, I couldn't help but notice that this blanket was conspicuously bowed upward.  No, the 18-year-old patient wasn't pregnant—she was simply obese, although "simply" seems a tad understated when we're talking about 275 pounds on a 5'1" frame.  I often get a gut feeling about certain things, and my gut feelings about her were on target.  In a split second, I'd guessed that she was a smoker, unemployed, and—of course—on welfare.  I also guessed that this was no emergency.  Such uncanny insights.

**Dr. Pezzi:**  What brought you into the emergency room today?

**Patient:**  The ambulance.

**Dr. Pezzi:**  (I thought, "Oh, we're a smart aleck, too, eh?")  *Why* did you come in?

**Patient:**  I've been having chest pain for two weeks.

**Dr. Pezzi:**  *Two weeks?*

**Patient:**  Well, maybe three . . .

**Dr. Pezzi:**  Have you seen your doctor about these pains?

**Patient:**  No, not yet.

**Dr. Pezzi:**  (Thinking, "Well, what are you waiting for?")  Why did you decide to come in today?

**Patient:**  'Cause me and my boyfriend are going on a trip tomorrow.  He got his disability check today, and we're going to the Mega-Mall to go shopping.

**Dr. Pezzi:**  (Musing, "No wonder my taxes are so high!")  Did you come to the ER because your pain is getting worse?

**Patient:**  No, it's getting better, actually.

*(Add another $2000 to the national debt.  A bevy of tests later, I had CYAed her to the max, even though I knew I would find nothing*[16]*.  To an*

---

[16]    At this juncture, it would be reasonable to ask, "Well, if you *knew* the tests would be negative, why did you order them?"  A good question deserves a good answer, and I have one.  In this case, the patient had done nothing more serious than pull one of her chest muscles.  It took me about 10 seconds to unravel that mystery, and I could have been on to see my next patient, or to hold the hand of the grandmother who was dying of lung cancer in the next room—but no, I had to play the CYA game.  In this country, there are *far too many* malpractice

attorneys out for blood.  These prostitutes don't care if you're right; if you haven't provided concrete substantiation of your diagnosis, they will make you pay for their next Rolls-Royce. "But," you interject, "if you're right, she doesn't have a serious problem, so nothing will happen to her, so she can't sue you."  Oh, if life were only that simple!  The patient was a smoker; smokers are prone to blood clots; blood clots can travel to the lung, causing a pulmonary embolism (PE)—*and kill!*  This patient had other traits which heightened the risk of a PE, such as morbid obesity and a sedentary lifestyle.  She was planning on taking a long automobile trip to another state the next day, which substantially increased the chance of clot formation.  (It doesn't matter that the risk of a PE, even in this person, is relatively unlikely in the near future. I see so many thousands of patients in one year it is inevitable that some are going to develop serious problems, or die.)  **If she indeed had nothing *but* a pulled muscle on the day I saw her in the ER, but she developed a clot the next day, then died, what do you think would happen?**  Her family would point their fingers at me, and unleash a rapacious lawyer.  He would scream, "She had the clot on the day she saw you, and you said she just had a pulled muscle!  You let her die!  Now, sign the check."  And you know what?  In this screwed-up country, I would have to sign his million-dollar check, out of fear that the original O.J. jury, now free to pursue other interests, would award the family a few million more.  Now do you get my drift?  Even if she did *not* have the clot when I saw her, I couldn't prove it—so I would pay dearly, even though I was 100% correct.  When a person comes (or, in this case, rolls) into the ER, there's one more entrant into the Malpractice Lottery.  The fact that I see a patient in the ER is enough to make me potentially liable for any adverse event which might befall this person in the future.  That's why I grit my teeth when an obese, chain-smoking fast-food addict waddles into the ER:  I can diagnose them correctly, but if they die in the near future—and there's often a good chance of that—it's not a *natural death*, brought on by slovenly habits and outright stupidity, it's *malpractice*, or so it will be alleged.  Spin the wheel, write the check.  Do you know what it is like to be charged with something that you know you're innocent of?  It's enough to put you in a bad mood for a few years, I'd say.  And how will this make you eye your next patient, who might be your next lawsuit?  With distrust, extreme wariness, and—of course—a heaping dose of CYA.  I'm tired of playing this game; how about you?

Ironically, in the years to come, there will be increasing justification for malpractice lawsuits, because future doctors will be less intelligent than the doctors of today, and hence more likely to botch things up.  *What, did Pezzi say that?*  Bear with me for a moment; it makes sense.  Society has made it incredibly difficult to become a doctor.  The average physician has an I.Q. of 130, which might not sound very impressive when compared to *everyone's* average of 100—but just take a gander at the intelligence bell-curve histogram, and see how far up the ladder this is.  Way up, as in borderline genius.  Not bad for raw material, eh?  But this is but one prerequisite, society deems.  Now, take your youth, and devote it not to having fun, but to cramming an ungodly amount of information between your ears.  And, as compensation for this torture, you get to *pay for it!*  A would-be doctor must either have rich parents, or an incredible tolerance for debt, 'cause med school ain't cheap.  Then, finally, you're a doctor.  *Is it over yet?*  Not quite—it's just beginning.  You become a resident, and work 110 hours a week for an hourly wage that's two steps below that of a trainee at McDonald's®! You're a good decade away from your last real pleasure, and you haven't seen your Mom in ages.  Your best friends think you've died, and your girlfriend . . . uh, where is she, anyway? She's left you to be with someone with a semblance of a normal life.  That's what you have given up to become a doctor—a normal life, a fun life.  Then, you're out.  You're the fabled "real" doctor; that is, a doctor with a license to practice medicine.  Gee whiz, after all that, you might think someone would trust your professional opinion, but no.  Vultures, schooled as Monday-morning quarterbacks, are there to tell the jury that you're wrong, even when *you were right*.  Such an enjoyable game!  Now, who wants to play?  Increasingly, bright people, being bright, are saying *"No, thanks!"* to medicine, and are putting their intellectual gifts to other uses.  It doesn't take a genius to realize that such an eventuality will cause a decline in the I.Q.

**97**

*attorney, my professional opinion means little; he wants proof, so I give it.)*

**Dr. Pezzi:** (While the history, physical, and tests supported a benign diagnosis, I began to counsel the patient on things she could do that would reduce her risk of serious health problems, such as losing weight, giving up cigarette smoking, and exercising.)

**Patient:** I don't like to exercise.

**Dr. Pezzi:** Why?

**Patient:** It makes me tired.

**Dr. Pezzi:** Have you tried dieting?

**Patient:** I tried it once, but I got hungry. My Mom always said I was a big eater. She says I've got big bones.

**Dr. Pezzi:** (Thinking, "No one's bones are *that* big!") It's very important that you stop smoking and lose weight. Otherwise, you will eventually develop serious problems.

**Patient:** *So what?*

**Dr. Pezzi:** Aren't you concerned about these risks to your health?

**Patient:** No. When I die, I die. I don't care *when* I die, as long as I can do whatever I want while I'm alive.

Hmmm . . . Fair enough. Everyone is entitled to their own opinion, especially on that matter. However, I wondered, if that is your opinion, **why** did you come to the ER *by ambulance*—wasting thousands of dollars—when you have no intention of following medical advice? For a moment, I began to mull over the "*why*," but my thoughts were interrupted.

**Patient:** Will you *get out of here?*

---

of future doctors. As I mentioned above, the *average* med student I.Q. is 130, but there are a good number of medical students with I.Q.s of 140, 150, 160, and even higher. The question is not what *can* they do, but what *can't* they do? The answer is, not much. They certainly don't need medicine to make a decent, *tolerable* living—they can go to work for Bill Gates at Microsoft and become a millionaire in a few years, and not have some shyster cant to the jury, "*He's wrong, he's wrong, he's wrong.*" Diverting bright people away from medicine will either result in many empty seats in the medical school lecture halls, or it will result in future doctors being less intelligent—and hence, less capable—than current doctors. Do you really want a neurosurgeon with an I.Q. of 110 poking around inside your head? I didn't think so. If the current trends continue, you won't have much of a choice. *Someone* has to pick up the scalpel and play brain surgeon, right Jethro? If the bright people are all working at Microsoft, you're out of luck.

**Dr. Pezzi:** (Startled, I thought, "Excuse me for intruding in *your* emergency room!") Pardon me?

**Patient:** Come on, *hurry up!* My boyfriend wants to talk to me about our trip tomorrow!

**Dr. Pezzi:** (Miffed, I *felt* like saying, "OK, you insolent blimp, I'll leave." However, I doubted that she'd know the meaning of "insolent," so the implication would be lost. I turned around, paused for a moment, and left. On to my next patient.)

■ Sitting at my desk in the ER, taking a well-deserved break from attending to a seemingly unending series of wacky patients, I looked up at the nurse, who slowly walked toward me while shaking her head from side to side. From the scornful look on her face, I knew that she was disgusted with the next patient, whose chart she handed to me as she rolled up her eyes. "She popped a pimple."

Incredulously, I responded, "What? She came to the emergency room because she *popped a pimple?*"

Smiling disdainfully, she said, "Yes. She scratched her back, and she popped a pimple. That's it." I thought to myself, "This must be *some* pimple." Well, ol' Doc Pezzi has to see that pimple. I trudged into her room, expecting to find a huge, festering sore that would be better termed an *abscess* than a *pimple*.

Initially, at least, I wasn't disappointed. The patient was smiling and surprisingly cute, and she had on a dressing so large that one might guess that she'd been struck by an artillery round. I felt relieved that this visit was justifiable, but this sense of relief was short-lived. Peeling off the dressing, I was greeted by a pimple so small that it wouldn't pique the interest of a dermatologist, let alone an *emergency* physician. There, in all of its glory, was a small (actual size = •) pimple that was amazingly lacking any signs of surrounding infection or other complications.

Why, I inquired, did she come in for this problem? She responded, "It was bleeding." Well, pimples have a habit of doing that when they're popped. However, in the entire history of the world, the number of people who have bled to death from popping a pimple is . . . *can you hold the flash card a little higher, Johnnie? . . .* uh, *zero!* Even if I multiplied the estimated blood loss by a factor of 10, her blood loss was about 1.5 cc, or less than one-third of a teaspoon. Thankfully, I passed my ATLS (Advanced Trauma Life Support) course with flying colors!

# Annals of Cause & Effect

**J-17**    Thursday, November 8, 2029    *The Detroit Times-News-Star-Gazette-Journal*

## Medical/Professional

### ATTENTION ALL MASOCHISTS!

*Want to be a doctor?* Apply to medical school now. Fall classes start in two weeks, but plenty of vacancies remain. If you've attended college (or at least attended a few college football games), and can tie your shoes correctly most of the time, you meet our ever-declining standards of admission. After paying $375,000.00 tuition per year for four years, we will foist you into the real world, where you'll receive the following benefits:

• *Call yourself Doctor!* Nobody else will, but what the heck?
• Money, money, money $$$. Like to write checks? *Good!!* You will be writing checks to pay off your student loans every month until you're 98 years old.
• Love attention? You will get plenty! Congress, insurance companies, state medical boards, irate patients, countless medical committees, and lawyers galore will give you lots of attention. Enjoy!
• Want a challenge? No matter what you do, someone will find fault with it. If you like being wrong, you're in for the time of your life.
• Crave thrills? Although a cure for AIDS was discovered in 2003, the Ebola VI virus, easily transmissible from infected patients, will guarantee that every day will be special—*and maybe your last!*
*DON'T DELAY, APPLY TODAY!!*

## Miscellaneous

### ANTIQUE SNOWMOBILE SHOW

Rare opportunity to view machines that traveled on snow—back in the days when there *was* snow, before global warming really took hold. Open 10 A.M. - 9 P.M. Saturday & Sunday at Cobo Hall. Tickets $25 at the door; also available on the Internet at oh.no.no.snow.com.

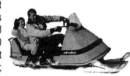

### FREE PUPPIES!

AKC registered, certified diet never fed Mad Cow Chow. Housebroken and wormed. Call 555-9362 eve. after 6.

### HOUSE FOR SALE

Northern Michigan. 3476 sq. ft., lower level walk-out finished basement. Robotic vacuum and lawn mower. 5 bedrooms, 3 baths, and gizmos too numerous to mention. Constructed circa 1994. McGovern Realty 555-4102. By appointment only.

### COMPUTER

Intel 4000 MHz P-38. 500 Gb RAM, 9048 x 6200 display. C
555-8395 after 4.

### ROCKET BELT

Used once.
555-7171

It's 1998
The golden age of medicine
has passed. Think it is bad to
be a doctor now? Wait another 3
years or so. In the realization that the
grass *is* greener on the other side of the
hill, intelligent people will shun medical school
As the intelligence of applicants drops, admissions
committees will either lower their standards, or have a
number of empty seats in the lecture hall
Taken far enough . .

Remembering the three-for-one rule, I mused, "What should I do, start an IV and give her a teaspoon of fluid?" Oh, I was being my usual silly self, alright, but—*come on*—who would deem such a problem an emergency? Common sense would dictate that this was no emergency. So, why come to the ER? I was about to find out, and the answer would leave me reeling in disbelief.

Batting my head as I exited the room of the pretty pimple-popper, the nurse inquired, "Well, did you *find* it?" I said that I had, but I was shocked that she came in for something so trivial. "Didn't you know," she asked, "that the government actually reimburses mileage for some Medicaid recipients when they drive to an ER?" I hadn't. "Yes, they do. Sometimes they will just 'stop by' when they're in town, so that they will be paid for the drive." I was dumbfounded. I knew that legislators often prostitute themselves when they steal the taxpayers' money, and hand it over to Medicaid recipients in the hope that these recipients will return the favor with a quid pro quo vote during the next election, but I had no idea that politicians would be so feeble-minded as to encourage and reward people for wasting precious health care dollars. But the name of the game is scratch my back, and I'll scratch yours. Even if it does pop a pimple.

■ "Welcome to the ER! Come one, come all, for a problem that is big, or a problem that is small." Hoping to increase ER revenue, hospital administrators and their underlings encourage ER personnel to make every ER patient feel welcome, regardless of whether the problem is serious and legitimate, or wacky and inane. At a time when perspicacious people are seeking ways of curtailing health care expenditures, hospital administrators are doing everything possible to loot the U.S. Treasury and health insurance companies. In the short-term, it is advantageous for the hospital to pillage the system, but in the long-term, such behavior is shortsighted, perpetuating and exacerbating a problem that affects every American either directly, or indirectly by dampening the U.S. economy. The need to economize is an altruistic imperative which demands the attention of everyone. When hospital administrators repudiate such a concern, it is morally and functionally equivalent to counterfeiting. This problem persists because very few people who deliver health care have the courage to stand up and say to patients whose ER visits are inappropriate, "This isn't an emergency. You don't belong in an ER." Instead, afraid of being sued[17], afraid of incurring the wrath of the administrators, afraid of

---

[17]     Concerned about the one-in-a-zillion chance the B.S. problem could somehow be linked to the eventual development of a problem that might result in a lawsuit, and concerned that any disparagement of the original concern might serve as self-righteous ammunition for the plaintiff's attorney, healthcare personnel are hesitant to suggest that any problem, no matter

the eternal dread of offending anyone, ER personnel usually remain silent, or—even worse—actively participate in this fiscal prostitution. "Yes! Glad you're here! You have a mosquito bite? A loose vagina? You've been farting? Popped a pimple? Have a problem that eludes diagnosis by the doctors at the Mayo Clinic[18]? Happy to ~~rape the system~~, uh, happy to serve you!"

■ A 29-year-old man walked into the ER at 7:45 a.m., complaining of a sore throat he'd had for the past day. He was given the option of being seen immediately in the ER, or waiting 15 minutes until the emergency department clinic opened at 8:00 a.m. He was told the clinic charge would be considerably less than the regular ER charge. Given that this guy didn't even look sick, let alone in any distress, I assumed he'd do the logical thing and wait 15 minutes. Wrong. He wanted to be seen immediately, so the bill went from $60 to something in the hundreds. In my mind, this is an inexcusable, all-too-typical indifference to health care cost containment. Was it *truly* worth a few hundred dollars to be seen 15 minutes sooner? I don't think so. On exam, the manifestations of his infection were definitely present, yet on the milder end of the sore throat spectrum.

After the exam, as I was writing a prescription for this fellow, he began complaining about the cost of his health insurance. Since this man seemed to be of average intelligence, I was struck by his failure to appreciate the correlation between his behavior and high health insurance premiums. Such a mystery.

Mrs. N. was a kindred spirit. She brought her previously-ill daughter to the ER at 7:20 a.m., saying that she had *had* a cold, but seemed much better now. Is this what emergency rooms are for? The child was happy, smiling, and obviously no longer ill. She mentioned that her child had an

---

how wacky, might not justify a visit to the ER. Every day, every hour, I see patients who say in so many words, "I have a serious problem. This is a lawsuit if you ignore this complaint." Yet, I know it's either 100% bull$#!+, or dramatically and unjustifiably magnified for effect, so I internally trivialize the complaint, and externally launch into well-practiced CYA banter. Consider, for example, the mother who brought her child to the ER because the kid received *one* mosquito bite. The child had no history of any problems with mosquito bites, and he had no problem with this bite. He had a tiny little bump on his skin, "Yup, looks like a mosquito bite." To put this in eloquent medical terminology, *BFD!* If everyone who sustained a mosquito bite came to the ER each time they were bitten, there would be a ten mile-long line of people waiting to get into the ER. Sure, there is an infinitesimally small chance of a complication developing as a result of a mosquito bite, but it is *insane* to go to the ER for such a problem. Even if the cost of the visit is ignored, a person faces a greater risk of death driving to and from the ER than he does from the bite itself.

[18]     To those readers who haven't read the rest of this book: these problems spurred actual patients to come to the ER. The woman with the loose vagina, you might recall, came in *by ambulance*. How ludicrous!

appointment with her pediatrician at 9:00 a.m. that morning, for the same questionable reason that caused her to come to the ER that morning: to be told her daughter was over her cold. This was ludicrously obvious.

What was more difficult to understand was why Mrs. N., given her low threshold of seeking medical attention, did not want her son to be evaluated by either the ER or their pediatrician. The son, who accompanied his sister to the ER, was clearly ill, with a cough so congested it made *my* chest rattle every time he began hacking. I commented on the cough, wondering if the Mom wanted me to examine her son, but her thoughts were elsewhere. "Darn it! I knew it! She's over her cold, and now I'm going to be stuck with a bill for both the emergency room *and* the pediatrician!" (She was still going to take her daughter to the pediatrician? The answer was yes.) Continuing on, as I recoiled in disbelief, she said, "And I had to get myself and the kids up early today, so that we could come into here! I bet the insurance company won't pay for this!" (I bet she's right.) "You doctors charge too much! Do you know how much I spend on doctor bills?" (I have no idea, but—in view of her level of common sense—I wouldn't be easily surprised.) "Someone ought to do something about doctor and hospital bills!" (It's always the other guy, right?)

As my shift ended at 8 a.m. and I walked out of the hospital, I smiled. It was good to be back in the world of sanity.

But not for long. As I entered the emergency department 12 hours later, I was greeted by chatter emanating from the speakerphone on the emergency radio. And, from the pained look on the face of the nurse who was listening to the incoming report, it was clear that she knew something I didn't know, and she was not very happy. "Oh, shit," she lamented, "she was just here! She was admitted for five days, and they didn't find anything wrong with her. She was discharged *this morning*!" Yikes, I thought, that either means **1)** the doctors missed something, or **2)** she was having a serious new problem, or a marked exacerbation of the old problem, or **3)** she didn't belong in an ambulance **or** an ER **or** a hospital. Experience told me that the answer was option #3. When the patient arrived 15 minutes later, it was *me* who was saying, "Oh, shit." It was #3, alright.

The "patient" (I'm using that term quite loosely, since she would be better described as a *visitor*) was a 71-year-old lady who'd been having chest pain for 18 years. That is not a misprint; it wasn't 18 minutes, hours, days, weeks, or months—it was 18 years! The pain was no different, she told me, but she was frustrated that they hadn't yet discovered the cause of it, and she wanted to be admitted once more. I wondered if she was suffering from the delusion that such a readmission would actually be fruitful, or if she possessed a secret addiction to hospital food. Having tasted the slop that passes for food at this institution, I doubted the latter. Her husband was no less adamant. "You've got to admit her! I can't take care of her at home!" I've heard that shenanigan before, and there is usually a grain of truth in it. But not this time. From his statement, you might infer that his wife was a tottering, frail, bedridden woman, but this was hardly the case. She was spry, intelligent, and attractive enough for her age (and she certainly didn't *look to be 71*) to appear in a Geritol® commercial. Physically, she was better off than many women half her age. "So," wonders the perpetually inquisitive Pezzi, "why *can't* he 'take care of her at home'?" She was also in a good mood, and was smiling and laughing as she and her husband debated the upcoming Presidential election. Some invalid, eh? Intensive care unit, here we come! Not quite.

Two thousand dollars of unremarkable tests later, I called the on-call physician for Internal Medicine. "$#!+*&@%, I discharged her a few hours ago! She has had every test in the world done on her! She has seen umpteen specialists! She has been tested at the Mayo Clinic! Why the heck is she here again?" I didn't have an answer for that. Flipping through the pragmatic lessons I've learned in my 10 years as an ER physician, though, I came across a few which seemed apropos.

> **Lesson #447:** People who smile and laugh do *not* have a serious cause of chest pain. I've seen a lot of people with a heart attack, and none of them have been in a joking mood. Ditto for the other serious causes of chest pain.

> **Lesson #448:** People who have unremitting chest pain for 18 years, and are still alive, do *not* have a serious cause of chest pain. A corollary to this is that such people who come in by ambulance are wasting a heap of money. The ambulance bills *alone* for her numerous "emergency" trips to the ER would buy a very nice home. Another corollary is that if people were responsible for their own medical expenses, this lady would be at home watching *Jeopardy*, not speeding to the ER in an ambulance.

Notwithstanding the veracity and applicability of my pragmatic postulates, the husband knew that I was going to discharge his wife from the ER, and he was mad. If he had a skewer, I'd probably be roasting over a pit by now. If his wife were to die in the near future (*hey, stranger things have happened to 71-year-olds!*), you can bet that he'd sue me for malpractice. To review: malpractice exists when you did something that an *average* physician of your same specialty would not do, **and** this error resulted in harm to your patient. Given that the best doctors in America couldn't come up with an explanation for her chest pain, it's not surprising that I didn't have a plausible diagnosis, either. But that would hardly dissuade an attorney from *alleging* malpractice; to them, malpractice = a bad outcome + let's scare the doctor into settling out-of-court. A bluff, no doubt, but one that works often enough to keep them eating caviar for breakfast. Yes, I'd probably "win" *this* case, but let me tell you what it's like to "win" . . .

■ It was 7:55 on a Sunday morning, and the doorbell rang. I wondered who was there. I didn't order a pizza yet, and I forgot to mail in my entry into the Publisher's Clearinghouse, so I was stumped. Who *was* there? I opened the door, and got my answer. Without even the most cursory social preface, the gruff visitor demanded, "Are you Dr. Pezzi?" Something told me that I'd soon wish I weren't, but I said that I was. With polished adroitness, he plucked a paper from his coat, and shoved it my way. "You're being sued. Have a nice day." Have a *nice day?* Being *sued?* Such a cruel oxymoron, I opined. Once my pulse fell below 160, I looked at the name of the plaintiff—you know, the person that I'd so heinously ravaged, who was suffering because of my egregious error. The name didn't ring a bell.

Sunday passed with precious little enjoyment, much to my utter surprise. On Monday, I drove to the hospital and examined the medical record of this patient. After scrutinizing every word of his chart, I was more puzzled than ever. Why *was* I being sued? The man had come to the ER with high blood pressure, and I'd placed him on intravenous medications to lower his blood pressure, which came down nicely. His evaluation in the ER was unremarkable, he felt great and took a snooze, and he was later admitted to the cardiology service and placed in one of our Intensive Care Units.

Why *was* I being sued? His hospital course was equally uneventful, and he was discharged the next week. Over the subsequent few months, he was seen in the cardiology clinic, where his blood pressure was carefully monitored. He was noted to be noncompliant with his medicine and prescribed diet, and he had not made the slightest effort to lose weight and stop smoking, but he was about as healthy as such a person could be. Why *was* I being sued? He then stopped going to the cardiology clinic, and began to see a physician in private practice. A few months after he began to see this physician, he had a questionable "heart attack," was treated for it, and resumed working, and resumed snorting cheeseburgers.

Again, why *was* I being sued? Even if I knew in advance that this patient would sue me, I couldn't have done anything any better. And, if I do say so myself, I did a superb job of CYA. Oh, but let's not forget the lawyer's strategy: bad outcome + doctor's fear of a Michigan jury = my wife's new

Mercedes-Benz. Conspicuously absent from that equation is any mention of a medical error, but such a trivial point would not deter an unscrupulous ~~prostitute~~, uh, attorney. If the plaintiff really wanted to sue the person responsible for his heart attack, he should have sued himself. But such a notion is contrary to the prevalent American tendency to disavow any culpability for a self-induced malady. Had about 4000 too many meals at the all-you-can-eat restaurant? Been smoking 2½ packs per day since you were 13? Do you rely upon beer commercials for your menu planning? Do you consider walking into McDonald's® to be your sole form of exercise? Your wife been frying your meals in lard? Had a heart attack? *Dang, it ain't your fault! It ain't your wife's fault! Heck, no! It's the doctor's fault! Yup, that's right, the doctor's fault! Let's sue the bastard! Let's get him out of bed before 8 a.m. on a Sunday[19], and scare the shit out of him! Darn it, let's make him pay! I've been wronged! I've been aggrieved! I'm gonna get even, and buy me that Cadillac® I've been dreaming about.* Let me truncate this self-righteous drivel, and say two things: anyone who buys into this logic is an idiot, and any lawyer who takes on such a case is an unprincipled thug.

Sure, I had malpractice insurance, but there was a nonrefundable $5000 deductible that was incurred every time a plaintiff entered the semifinals of the Malpractice Lottery. Now for the bad part. The letters, phone calls, subpoenas, depositions, and plain ol' grief, from countless lawyers, secretaries, judges, clerks, witnesses, and sundry "experts." While I pleaded with my attorney to get me out of this case, he said that I'd just have to ride it out for a while. *A while?* Two years later, I was *still* being harassed. I wasn't too surprised, though. My defense attorney doesn't get paid unless he's working, and if he could have gotten me dismissed from this suit in 15 minutes, he wouldn't be making much money. It's just a game, he told me. The more I learned about this "game," the more I realized he was right, but the less I liked it.

Finally, I'd had enough of this crap. I called my attorney, and said that I wanted out, pronto. He agreed that the case against me was without any merit[20], so he called the plaintiff's prostitute, and indicated that if he kept me in this suit any longer, I'd have a great case against him for *legal* malpractice. The case he had against me was nonexistent; a more

---

[19]    The timing of this legal notice was no mistake. Attorneys often coach their underlings as to when to serve the papers, so as to inflict the greatest psychological blow to the defendant. One of the few attorneys that I like told me that he has, in a very calculated fashion, even served people on *Christmas Eve!* And this man is a decent fellow. Do law schools give courses in dishing out cruelty?

[20]    Other physicians who had treated this patient were also being sued, but this did little to console me.

frivolous lawsuit was inconceivable. Scared, he backed down. He "let me go." I was "free." I was "victorious." I had "won."

*Some victory!* It cost me $5000, one girlfriend, about 600 nightmares, and untold other hours of anguish. This fiasco was ongoing at the time I was applying for a new mortgage on my home, and the mortgage company routinely inquired if I was involved in any pending lawsuits. Since I was, I ended up paying a higher interest rate. OK, the suit was over. Did the mortgage company lower my interest rate now that I'm not being sued? "No," they told me, "but you're welcome to apply for a new mortgage, though." Thanks, I'll pass—I'd rather have all of my teeth pulled, without anesthesia. The $5000 was long gone, the nightmares were still reverberating in my mind, and I'd come to view almost every ER patient as a potential lawsuit. So much for my Marcus Welby image of becoming friends with my patients. And my girlfriend? Married, but not to me. Yes, I'd won. You still want to apply to medical school? This, mind you, was a *victory*.

Given that the allegations against me were totally unfounded, and given that I had suffered emotionally and economically from this baseless slander, I should have been able to sue the shyster, right? If a man walks up to you on a street, holds you at gunpoint, robs you of $5000-*plus*, and mashes your psyche, he is guilty, and can be sued for civil damages—*if* he is not an attorney, who is legally entitled to mercilessly plunder at will, with little or no fear of sustaining any personal repercussions. One-way battles are difficult to lose, and attorneys have stacked the deck quite nicely in their favor. Who permits such legalized rape[21]? The Congress, state legislatures, and the courts, which are primarily filled with—*can you guess?*—lawyers! Surprise, surprise. And when it comes to political payoffs, uh, donations, who is the staunchest supporter of these people? No surprise there: attorneys! A more perfect system of legislated piracy has yet to be invented.

And now, dedicated to the extinction of the politically empowered pretorian prostitutes who perpetuate such an unjust system, I offer the following musical interlude:

---

[21]    I am *not* being flip in my choice of words. When I say "rape," I mean it, with all of its literal meaning.

    Given my derision of this system, you might be surprised that I, as a patient, have been a victim of malpractice, too. This occurred when I was a teenager, and the thought of suing the doctor never even entered my mind.

# Malpractice? *Not by a mile!*

(Sung to the tune of *Gilligan's Isle*)

Just sit right back and you'll hear a tale,
A tale of an ER trip.
That started with a Blue Cross® card,
And ended with an alleged malpractice slip.

The patient was having a heart attack,
His wife was adamantly sure.
$3000 they spent that day,
On a 4-hour ER tour . . . a 4-hour ER tour.

The CYA game was essential stuff,
The doctor had to be sure.
If not for these defensive medical tests,
This could be a potential malpractice lure ... a potential malpractice lure.

The patient did well for many months,
But the lawyer still filed suit,
With allegations . . . of malpractice, too.
The plaintiff wants to be . . . a millionaire!
"This Lotto is sure fun!",
Says the hired gun.
Here—it's a one-way fight!

So this is the tale of a malpractice suit,
It'll be here for a long, long time.
They'll claim all sorts of damages,
The lawyer, he will chime.

The Congress and their cohorts, too,
Will do their very best,
To make the doctors miserable;
This they'll say without jest:
"No cell phone, no lights, no motorcar,
Take all of his luxuries!
Like Robinson Crusoe,
Make him as penniless as can be!"

So join us in Circuit Court, my friends,
I'm sure that you won't smile.
'Cause you're also paying for this,
And you've been for quite a while!

OK, let's go back to my original question: why was I sued? Certainly, there was no medical malpractice in this case. Apparently, the plaintiff's pea-brained attorney thought that since there are more drugs to lower blood pressure than the two which I administered, that I should have given him even more drugs. If two are good, five are better, right? Obviously not. There's such a thing as lowering blood pressure too much, and low blood pressure can be more dangerous than high blood pressure. Had the patient received all of the drugs suggested by his attorney, I agree that he would have had a different outcome: he would have been dead.

This attorney is clearly incompetent, both medically and legally. It doesn't matter that he's wrong and I'm right. It doesn't matter that I did an above-average job for this patient, whose blood pressure reduction was perfect. It doesn't matter that the questionable heart attack occurred several months after I'd treated him. If I, as an emergency doctor, could reasonably guarantee that every patient I've treated would not have a heart attack in the next year, they wouldn't call me "Doctor," they'd call me "God." Since I'm clearly not the latter, I think the standard of care to which I'm being held is ludicrous. But this is America, the land in which the legal profession has warped the concept of justice so radically that innocent people can be terrorized with impunity. Their tactics are simple: drive a wedge between the general population and the targeted group, disparaging them as being the root of societal problems, thus creating an "us-versus-them" mentality in the minds of the masses. Then, when the leaders say "attack," the masses mindlessly comply. Is this America? Or is it at least vaguely reminiscent of another country that was notorious for its internal terrorism? While the evil thus engendered is incomparably disparate, their tactics bear an execrable similarity, and they are both plainly reprehensible.

While I know that physicians occasionally make egregious errors for which they should be held accountable, I fail to understand why society places such a singular burden of personal liability upon doctors. To illustrate this disparity, let's consider the case of two professionals who are judging whether or not a certain person is a danger to society. Assume that both professionals concluded the person was not a danger to others, and could be released. If the person were released and murdered someone, there is a strong likelihood that the professional would be sued if he were an emergency physician. On the other hand, if the professional were a judge, he would be immune to a suit for alleged malpractice. If the judge wished, he could adjourn the court and postpone his decision until he had given it a great deal of thought, and obtained the opinions of a number of experts (and called the Psychic Hotline, if he so desired). On the other hand, an ER physician may have to make such a determination within minutes, without benefit of ancillary support, all the while enmeshed in the chaos of the emergency department. Notwithstanding these factors, society allows physicians to be sued for millions of dollars in such cases, but judges get off scot-free. Given the circumstances in which they work, it would be more logical to excuse the error of the harried ER doctor, and to penalize the unhurried judgement of the judge. But that's the exact opposite of the extant laws. Such a chasm of accountability underscores the fact that justice is not evenly dispersed.

Another ludicrous disparity in professional accountability concerns the private lives of physicians vis-à-vis judges or attorneys. I recently read in the newspaper that a certain physician faces up to life in prison (!!) because he had sex with a patient. If he raped her, or if she were not an adult, such a sentence would be understandable. But she was a consenting adult[22] who met him in various out-of-town motels for trysts. For this the doctor should be penalized with a life sentence? *It's insane!* The punishment is far worse than the crime—*if* there was any crime at all (heck, murderers usually get off easier!). If a judge or an attorney slept with a defendant, it would make for quite a scandal, but they would never face the prospect of imprisonment for life.

■ Even by ER standards, this patient was out of control. After downing what could only be termed an excessive amount of alcohol, she forgot to pick her child up from school. This was apparently not the first time this had happened, so the principal paid her a visit, and wisely chose to bring along the state police. Good idea. This woman didn't take kindly to visitors appearing so early in the day (4 p.m.), so she began throwing furniture at them. Her hospitality left something to be desired, but her fighting skills did not, so it took an additional police unit or two to subdue her. That accomplished, the police brought her to the ER for evaluation.

*Why?* Why bring her to the ER? What's the emergency? Because she's 2½ times the legal limit of intoxication? (This level, incidentally, is so common in ER patients that it wouldn't raise an eyebrow.) Because she was vicious and not easily tractable? Because she reveled in her turpitude? Because her punch packed one heck of a wallop, as I later found out?

---

22    The patient now contends that she felt pressured into having sex with the physician because, she alleges, he said that he would not continue to be her physician unless she consented to have intercourse with him. Thus, the prosecutor contends, this is tantamount to coercion. What a specious argument! Even if the allegation were true, anyone with a room-temperature I.Q. would realize that coercion could not be effected in such a manner. Let's see . . . my doctor won't continue treating me unless I consent to intercourse, and that's not something I want . . . oh, what *should I do?* This is obviously not one of the great mysteries of the Universe. The answer is simple: fire the guy, and get another doctor. *Duh!*

*Answer*: none of the above. The reason she was brought to the ER is that police fear lawyers almost as much as doctors do. Once in a blue moon, there's a drunk whose kookiness is caused by a medical problem. So, to avert later allegations that they overlooked something, the police bring these wackos to the ER.

If you have never witnessed the ruckus these nuts can stir up, you're lucky. Their profanity could make a sailor blush, and their outbursts could make George Foreman run for cover. Their behavior in the ER can be so unspeakably noxious that I've seen patients with legitimate emergencies skedaddle out of the ER. The ones who stay pay the price. Babies cry, grandmothers hold their hands over their ears, and grown men wince in disgust. The police don't *want* to bring this riffraff to the emergency room; 99.99% of the time, they know who needs to be in an ER, and who just needs to be behind bars. But in America, it's lawyers who pull the strings. Similar to the dilemma that doctors often find themselves in, it is simply not good enough for the officer to be correct. If the kook did *not* have a medical problem at the time, but later developed one, the police would have no proof of this. Some unscrupulous lawyer, salivating at the chance to make a quick buck (or 400,000 of them), would gleefully allege that the police threw the criminal in jail, when he should have been resting in a nice, comfy hospital bed. Given the propensity of criminals to sue, and given the inherent difficulty in defending such cases, the police do the only logical thing: bring the riffraff to the ER.

In addition to creating the above-mentioned turmoil, the obvious need for thoroughly CYAing these cases merely adds another burden onto the backs of the taxpayers. In the past decade, I've never seen one prisoner with a problem that would not have been obvious to a layman. Many prisoners have *claimed* that they're having a heart attack, stroke, or other serious malady, but—zillions of CYA dollars later—not one case has panned out. I'm opposed to such low-yield testing. However, doctors must choose between bankrupting the taxpayers, or facing the possibility of personal bankruptcy resulting from a malpractice suit. Naturally, they choose the former; you'd do the same, too.

This gloomy situation will persist unless there is a fundamental change in the ideology of the politicians who are elected to the higher echelons of government. Current politicians, who have a vested interest in preserving the status quo, have repeatedly demonstrated their reluctance to enact laws which would obviate the need for doctors (and police) to be so defensive. Let your politicians know that you're fed up with their harping on nauseatingly nebulous "issues" such as "family values." Tell them that you want more of your paycheck in *your* pocket, instead of being diverted into defensive CYA posturing. Malpractice reform can get the lawyers off *your* back, and out of *your* wallet.

■ Rob was an all-too-frequent visitor to the ER. Each time I saw him, I couldn't believe that he'd have the temerity to perpetuate his charade. He claimed to have back pain, for which he demanded narcotics. In the ER, he'd hobble around as if he were crippled, occasionally shedding a fake tear or two when he thought that might garner a sympathetic prescription. He didn't know that we would watch him after he left the ER, though. Once he was through the doors, he would briskly walk toward his brand-new Corvette convertible (incidentally, he was on Medicaid), and hop in it without even bothering to open the door. Yup, that poor fella must have been having some terrible back pain.

Eventually, we learned that Rob wasn't his real name. He was using so many aliases that it must have been confusing to him, trying to keep his lies straight. After I learned one of his other names, I decided to trick him. I walked into his room and said, "Hi Steve, how are you doing? You look like you're in a lot of pain. Can I get you something for it, Steve?"

"Oh yeah, thanks Doc."

If someone called me "Fred" twice within ten seconds, I'd certainly mention to them that I'm not Fred. Especially in a hospital. But Rob said nothing. Hmmm . . .

Among his repertoire of skills was a semi-competent talent for forging or altering prescriptions. I say "semi-competent" because he made some egregious errors which drew the pharmacist's attention, such as spelling "capsules" incorrectly. There aren't too many doctors out there who spell it "capsilles."

Early one morning, Rob was in the ER, once again requesting a prescription for narcotics. But he made another blunder: he asked me to hand him his jacket, which I did. When I lifted the jacket, it felt weighted down, and there was the unmistakable sound of pills rattling in a bottle. *Several* bottles. Knowing Rob as I did, I assumed they were narcotics. "Hey, Rob, what do you have in your pockets?"

"N-n-n-nothing," he slurred. Although it was only 7 a.m., it was clear to me that he was already doped up.

I shook his jacket up and down a few times, rattling the pills loudly. Dang, there must be hundreds of pills in there. "Sure doesn't sound like *nothing* to me," I said.

"T-t-t-that's none of your business!"

"Oh, I think it is my business. If a patient is requesting a narcotic prescription, I think it is important for me to know what other pills he is taking. I wouldn't want any of my patients to *overdose*, you know."

"Y-y-y-you can't look in my pockets! Gimme that jacket!"

"You're right—I can't legally search your jacket. On the other hand, there's no law which says that I have to be a fool and give you more narcotics. So I'll make you a deal. If you show me the pills, and if any of them are not narcotics or other controlled substances, I will consider helping you out."

"N-n-n-no way!" he screamed.

"Well, I never prescribe any medication for a patient without knowing the other medicine they're taking. Could be a harmful drug interaction. So I'm not going to write a prescription for you."

"Y-y-y-you're not a good doctor. I'm leaving!"

But not for long. He returned a few hours later and saw the physician working the day shift, who relented to Rob's incessant pressure and gave him a prescription for a narcotic. Rob left once more, this time quite pleased.

Wouldn't you know it? A few hours later, and he was back again. This time, however, he was brought to the hospital in an ambulance, unconscious from a drug overdose. When he awoke later on in the ICU, he signed himself out AMA (against medical advice) and left the hospital. He never came back. I assumed he'd learned his lesson—or finally died from his habit.

A few years later, after I moved to a different part of the state, I was working in the ER when he walked through the door. When he saw me, he startled briefly and then exclaimed, "Oh, no, not *you* again!" He immediately turned around and left. As he was leaving, I noticed that he was holding his Medicaid card. I also noticed that he was walking without difficulty. He hopped into yet another new Corvette, and sped off. The Medicaid fraud business must pay pretty well, I mused. Even I can't afford a Corvette.

# *Just a jerk*

■ ER physicians occasionally find themselves facing some wild, unsubstantiated accusations. For example . . .

While working in the ER one night several years ago, I was mired in a sea of bad protoplasm. To put it another way, I had a number of *sick* people on my hands. The gentleman in bed #1 was having a heart attack. The young lady in bed #2 had attempted to kill herself by taking a number of pills. The elderly man in bed #3 had also attempted to kill himself, and was brought to the ER by the police. He was comatose. The woman in bed #4 was flip-flopping through so many abnormal cardiac rhythms that she could have been the sole subject for an extremely advanced class in cardiac life support. The lady in bed #5 was in septic shock (meaning that she had a very bad infection which caused her blood pressure to plummet; this can be fatal). To complicate matters, she was also having a heart attack. And this was only in the first 5 beds! As usual, I was the only doctor on duty and other patients in the ER were clamoring about why they had not been taken care of. Then the fun began. The boyfriend of the patient in bed #2 had decided she did not require admission to the hospital, which I had earlier discussed with them. It is standard practice to admit people who attempt suicide. Apart from the medical reasons for admission, it is obvious that such people cannot receive enough counseling from the ER doctor so that their lives are miraculously and suddenly worth living once more. The boyfriend, however, informed me that his girlfriend was safe and would not try killing herself again. The boyfriend had no training in medicine or psychology, but knew he was right. I explained to him that it was impossible to conclude this with 100% assurance, and that she would require admission. An hour ago she tried to kill herself, and now he is positive she is OK? I don't buy it, and neither would her attorney if I were dumb enough to discharge her and she tried the same thing again.

Such logic failed to impress the boyfriend. After reiterating my position numerous times, I told him it was futile for him to attempt to sway my opinion. He walked away, and I resumed working. After a while, I noticed he was pestering the nurses with the same inane argument. They were embroiled in attempting to save the lives of several people, and anyone who was interfering with their work was literally contributing to murder. I'd had enough of this jerk. I told the nurses to ignore him, and I asked him to leave the ER as his behavior was endangering people's lives. He refused. I called security, and had him escorted out of the ER.

End of story? Nope. He felt I had violated his "civil rights," and turned me in to some civil rights commission. They investigated the matter, and found it had no merit. That was obvious. What surprised me was why the boyfriend felt justified in referring this matter to them in the first place. While he was black, the issue of race never came up in any manner while I was talking to him. Frankly, I never even thought of him as a black man—I just thought of him as a man who was endangering others by his behavior. I couldn't care if he were black or white. I value people by their actions, not by their color.

■ The ER nurse walked by me, casually announcing that the father of the child I'd just admitted would like to ask me some questions. The child had been brought in by his Mom, and the Dad had just arrived. I was curious as to why he wanted to see me, as I had been unusually thorough in explaining everything to the Mom, and I thought she could explain everything to him. After all, the case was not very complicated—the child had been run over by a tractor, but the tractor obviously didn't touch the kid, who fortuitously was positioned between the tire tracks. Physically, the child was fine, but the child's pediatrician wanted to play it safe and keep him overnight in the hospital for observation. After meeting the Dad, I knew why the pediatrician was being so cautious.

Taking his apparel cues—and perhaps the clothing itself—from a 1950s biker magazine, the Dad was dressed in a black leather suit, into which was ground enough dirt to make me wonder if he was planning to grow something on his suit, or if he just had a serious problem staying on his motorcycle. Sitting on a chair, he had his legs spread widely, and his head was jauntily cocked to the side and slightly backward. His face looked hardened and older than his years, though he was only 25 or so. His eyes glared at me with contempt and resentment, and his mouth was curled into a band of hatred. If looks could kill, I would have been dead. I'd met the Dad, and entered the realm of surly brusqueness.

**Dad:** So, what's wrong with the kid?

**Dr. Pezzi:** Nothing; he appears to be fine. He was quite lucky, you know.

**Dad:** Whatta ya mean, "lucky"?

**Dr. Pezzi:** I mean, if one of the tires had rolled over him, there's a good chance that it could have killed him.

**Dad:** How da ya know that?

**Dr. Pezzi:** Uh (caught off guard by such a silly question) . . . The tractor must weigh several thousand pounds.

**Dad:** So nothin' is broken?

**Dr. Pezzi:** Right.

**Dad:** Ya sure about that? When I was a kid, the stupid doctors said nothin' was wrong with me, and my foot was broken.

**Dr. Pezzi:** No, nothing is broken. If his foot were broken, your child wouldn't be able to walk so easily. (By this time, the kid had been dancing in the ER, bouncing around with so much energy that one might think that he was related to Richard Simmons.)

**Dad:** Nothin' better be broken, 'cause if it is, I'm comin' back in here!

**Dr. Pezzi:** Your son is OK.

**Dad:** What makes you think he ain't hurt?

**Dr. Pezzi:** The fact that he's smiling and playful, and running around the ER.

**Dad:** I'm tellin' ya right now, buddy, he'd better be fine . . .

OK, Cro-Magnon man, you've made your point, impressing me with your charm, and dazzling me with your brilliant wit and consummate verbal ability. *Sheesh!* Whatever happened to social pleasantries? Funny, no one ever spoke to Marcus Welby in such a manner. If I could go back to the time I was applying to medical school, I'd sing along with Johnny Paycheck, "Take this job and shove it . . ."

■ While I don't have virgin ears, there are times when I'm not willing to tolerate much profanity in the ER. On one particularly memorable night, Wayne seemed determined to expand my knowledge of profane words by the simple technique of repetition. Bellowing on and on, every sentence was littered with abusive insults, racial epithets, and a disgustingly large variety of swear words. His booming, water-buffalo voice echoed through the small emergency department. While I was not enjoying his performance, I was particularly concerned for the other patients in the ER at that time. A sweet little 4-year-old girl was literally feet from The Epicenter of Profanity (in that ER, every patient was within earshot of such a loudmouth). She required a few hours of monitoring in the ER before she was stable enough for admission, so she and her Mom were an unwilling but immobile audience. Other patients and their family members were similarly held captive. I tried appeasing Wayne, but he was not easily appeased. I tried cajoling him with the knowledge that his speech was upsetting the precious 4-year-old who was in the adjacent room, but he was not moved by such a request.

Eventually, a couple in their fifties left the ER, saying that they couldn't stand his outbursts any longer. I'd seen the man wincing as he heard Wayne cuss, and I tried every professional way I knew to put an end to this episode. When I lost a legitimate ER patient, I lost my patience. I walked into Wayne's room and grabbed the largest endotracheal tube (that's a tube which is inserted into a person's windpipe to facilitate breathing). Brandishing this in front of his mean, uncaring eyes, I explained that I was going to intubate him (that is, to insert the tube). Furthermore, I explained, I was going to do so via the nasotracheal route, which means that I was going to stick the tube into his windpipe by going through his nose. Once inserted, he would be unable to speak. Such a tragedy.

After a good second or two of reflection, Wayne backed down. Obviously dreading this possibility, he said, "OK, what do you want me to do?" I said that I wanted him to be quiet. He readily agreed to this, and he didn't utter a peep for the remainder of his stay in the ER. Surprised me, too.

Some of you may be wondering why I didn't put the hammer to Wayne sooner. In retrospect, I should have. However, I generally exhaust my conventional responses before resorting to threats. Admirably, some other ER physicians are not as tolerant of such behavior. When it's clear that they have such a rogue, recalcitrant patient, they will administer drugs to temporarily paralyze them, then they'll be intubated. Sometimes you have to fight fire with fire.

■ On another occasion, I had a unique weapon with which to combat unruly behavior. I'd seen Arnie in the ER a few months ago, at which time I'd inherited him from another physician who was leaving at the end of her shift. She asked me to check a certain lab test, and discharge him if that was OK. "Don't even bother to check him—he's just a drunk," she said. While I appreciated this timesaving tip, I am sufficiently anal that it meant nothing to me: I'd examine him, even if he were a foul-mouthed drunk.

At this visit, Arnie was complaining of abdominal pain. The second I palpated his belly, I knew why. His rigid abdominal wall indicated that his innards were being irritated, probably from a perforation of his bowels. To make a long story short, Arnie underwent surgery for just such a problem, and lived happily ever after.

Well, not this day. On this day, twenty or so weeks after his trip to the operating room, Arnie was in a particularly bad mood. At the time I arrived for the beginning of my shift, Arnie had been terrorizing the nurses for over an hour with his unique brand of profanity. Upon hearing his charming voice, I immediately devised a plan to put an end to his outbursts. Walking into his room, I said, "Hi Arnie! Remember me?" His sudden silence indicated that he had at least vaguely recalled who I was. Still, he said nothing. "I'm Dr. Pezzi. I saw you a few months ago when you had the ruptured bowels."

"Oh, yeah. That other doctor was going to send me home . . ."

"And I saved your life. So would you please do me a favor?"

"Sure, Doc, anything."

"Will you please stop harassing the nurses?" He did.

■ This event happened a few years before I began working in this ER. Fortunately for me. Someone—nobody knows just who, but it was presumably a disgruntled former ER patient—drove up to the ER entrance, and began firing a gun through its glass doors.

Wouldn't a complaint letter have sufficed?

■ Oh, great, another irate patient. Just what I need. Tom was brought to the ER by an ambulance after he slipped into a coma from a heroin overdose. I administered Narcan®, a drug which counteracts the effects of heroin and other opiates. Within minutes, Tom was awake. Darn.

"I want a refund!" he screamed.

"A *refund?*" I asked curiously.

"Yes, a refund! Do you know how much I paid for that heroin?"

"Nope."

"I paid a lot! And you wasted it! I ain't got no buzz from it, so I *demand* a refund!"

"Sorry to spoil your Saturday night, but I'm not going to give you any money for the dope."

"Then I'll sue your ass, just you wait and see!"

"I saved your life, Tom . . ."

"No, you wasted my money, and deprived me of my constitutional rights!"

"Your *constitutional* rights? Just what might they be?"

"My constitutional rights. I know I have them!"

"I didn't know there was a constitutional right to overdose on heroin."

"It's in there somewhere . . . the pursuit, the pursuit of . . . of . . ."

"Happiness?" I interjected.

"Yeah, that's it. You interfered with my constitutional right to the pursuit of happiness. You're in a heap of trouble, Mr. Doctor, violatin' my constitutional rights and all. You gonna pay for this!"

You can please some of the people all of the time, all of the people some of the time, but you can't please all of the people all of the time. Especially in an ER.

■ The Mom walked swiftly into the ER. Without saying a word or looking at anyone else, she handed me her baby. That's a bad sign. When a mother hands over her baby as if it's a hot potato, there's something seriously wrong with the child. When a child is very sick but isn't crying, that's an even worse sign. In this case, little Jessica wasn't breathing. Not bothering to excuse myself from the patient with head lice, I called for a nurse and we began resuscitating the baby.

As the infant's skin gradually changed from purple to pink, we all breathed a collective sigh of relief. When the baby awoke and began crying, we were all happy. The battle had been won. I'd have to address the underlying problem, but Jessica would live.

Well, *most* of us were happy. Clyde, the man with head lice, wasn't pleased with the delay in his treatment. He walked into Jessica's room and began complaining. "I'm tired of waiting. When the hell are you going to get back with me?"

The nurse was not pleased with this interruption. "You want to know when we're going to get back with you?"

"Damn right I do!"

"*Never!*"

■ The head nurse gingerly handed me a chart. "After you see this patient, Dr. Pezzi, please give the chart back to me. We're going to keep this chart separate from the others."

"Why is that?" I asked.

"She's threatening to kill one of the hospital vice-presidents. And she works here. She's the head of the accounting department." Not your run-of-the-mill patient, I mused.

After I saw the patient, I knew why she was mad. Her boss, the vice-president, was making unreasonable demands. He wanted her to fudge certain figures to create the illusion that his departments were fiscally better off than they actually were. Furthermore, the VP told her that if she were ever caught, he would deny knowing anything about it. If she refused to participate, he'd find some reason to fire her. Gee-whiz, and I'd thought that soap operas were purely fictional.

As she kept pounding her fist into the stretcher, tears of rage flowed down her face. "That S.O.B. only cares about advancing his own career!" she screamed. "I'll kill him!"

While I was no great friend of the VP, I was not anxious to see a gun battle in the hospital. I was afraid that innocent people might be injured, so I urged her to think of another means of resolving this conflict without having to resort to a consultation with Drs. Smith & Wesson.

"But how can I get out of this mess? He's got me. I'm darned if I do, and darned if I don't!"

"Sometimes you have to fight fire with fire," I explained.

"What do you mean by that?"

I explained what I would do in such a circumstance. "That's a great idea!" she exclaimed.

No, it wasn't. It backfired. Not against her—against me. The plan worked great from her perspective in that she was able to force the VP to back down and give up his illegal demands without creating any risk that she'd be fired. However, I never counted on the fact that she'd tell him that I was the source of her plan. From that day on, I was rather unpopular with the administration at that hospital. Had the VP known that I'd indirectly saved his life (she'd already procured the gun and the bullets), he probably would have had a better opinion of me. I never bothered to tell him, though.

■ Combine a dozen drinks with an overdose of cocaine, and mix it into an obnoxiously abrasive personality which just happens to be housed inside the body of a 26-year-old lawyer who thinks the world revolves around him. Combine these elements, and what do you get? A spark plug to ignite the ever-present latent volatility of the ER. This less-than-charming patient was brought to the ER by a couple of police officers, who pulled him over after seeing his car veer around the road. Todd was not pleased with this interruption of his evening plans. As I approached him, he screamed, "I'm a lawyer!!!"

I wondered if I should bow now, or later. "Yes?" I said.

"I'm a f------ lawyer! If you touch me, I'll sue you!"

"Well," I explained, "these police officers have a court order to obtain blood to determine if you've been driving under the influence of drugs or alcohol. I suppose it's that, or your driver's license will be automatically revoked."

"You're not touching me, and *no one* in here is touching me! Or I'll sue all of you! I love to sue people—it's what I do!"

The word "hyper" would not even begin to adequately convey the degree of his agitation. His speech was impressively rapid, and when he spoke he would thrust his trunk as far forward as his handcuffs would allow, with his face contorted in rage and spewing out a spray of saliva. Such professional decorum.

Since I was a rookie at the time of this incident, I wasn't sure where I stood on legal grounds. I called the judge who was on-call, and explained the situation to him. I also explained that I wanted to examine and treat the patient (not just draw his blood), as I was concerned he might have some medical complications from the cocaine. The judge gave me the authorization to do whatever I felt needed to be done, and he also told me to tell the lawyer to behave like a gentleman, or he'd have him disbarred. I liked that judge.

As I walked back to give him the good news, I saw that Todd had more company. The father of another patient had apparently had enough of Todd's foul mouth. This man, who could dwarf most NFL linebackers, was brandishing his fist in front of the face of Mr. Personality. The police officers seemed to enjoy his presence, as did I.

"You see this fist, loudmouth? Nobody uses language like that around my daughter! If you don't shut up, this fist is going to rearrange your face, got it?"

I liked that man, too, and I didn't charge him for his daughter's ER visit.

# Hold the pickles, hold the lettuce . . .

■ I'm puzzled. I've been working at a hospital which recently opened a larger ER. Hospital administrators, who presumably have some factual basis for their projection, gleefully predict that the new ER will attract 15% more "customers" than the old ER. This leaves me thinking, *"Why?"* It's not as if we opened a new restaurant with an expanded salad bar. In the area in which this hospital is located, it is, hospital-wise, in the middle of nowhere. Literally, it is not just the only game in town, so to speak, it is the only hospital in the county, and the only hospital serving several surrounding counties. So, if you have an emergency, you go there, regardless of whether or not you like the color of the paint on the walls. Why, then, should a new ER attract more patients? Will there be 15% more emergencies occurring in this community? Obviously not. Will patients drive a hundred miles just to be treated in a pretty ER? Not if they have a shred of common sense!

The only foreseeable explanation is that the 15% increase in patient volume will be filled from the ranks of the fringe-wacko patients, who come to the ER for incredibly obvious non-emergencies. Having an elegant new ER might entice them to forgo watching a few soap operas, and come to the ER to pester the staff with their inane complaints. As it is, the majority of ER patients don't belong in an ER, and a disgustingly large percentage don't need *any* sort of medical attention.

In the United States, our brilliant government has a rather potent law which legally obligates emergency rooms to provide care to anyone who walks in the door, regardless of their ability to pay, and regardless of how unjustifiably idiotic their complaint is. I've seen women come to the ER because they were dissatisfied with their perm. *What am I, a hairdresser?* Want a shampoo and blow-dry while we're at it? It's crazy, and you're paying for it! Aren't you glad you're working your butt off to pay for such bullshit? Let's tell the folks in Washington to wake up and put an end to their facilitation of this kind of behavior. Oh, no, better not ask them. If they did this, they might offend a portion of their constituency, and lose a few votes in the next election. Wimps.

■ Hospital administrators like to view patients not as *patients*, but as *customers*. Most of the higher echelon administrators have a background in business, not medicine. It shows. When I was around nine years old, my Dad gave me a list of good business principles, one of which was,

"The customer is always right." Administrators try to inculcate that concept into their medical and nursing staffs, hoping that the satisfied "customers" will come back, again and again.

In my mind, a *legitimate* patient is far more special than a customer. Walk into a store. "Will that be cash, check, or charge? Thank you for shopping here. Bye." Real special, aren't you? Your value as a customer to a businessman is proportional to the amount of money he can make off you. I'd be aghast if my doctor possessed that same mindset. Wouldn't you? Ah, but to an administrator, you're a potential source of revenue with a pulse. If you're a paying customer with good insurance or a fat wallet, they're glad to see you. If you're broke or have some cents-on-the-dollar insurance like Medicaid, they're not apt to smile. I've sat in on more than one meeting in which administrators brainstormed, trying to think of ways to bring in more "customers" with good insurance, while trying to subtly discourage Medicaid patients[23] and those who were unlikely to pay.

If you've read much of this book, you will know that I'm no fan of the Medicaid system. That attitude stems from repeated exposure to ER patients who had a Medicaid card but nothing which could be construed as an emergency, or even a medical problem. Having noticed that there is a correlation between the possession of a Medicaid card and the likelihood that the ER visit will be for some wacky, you've-got-to-be-kidding reason, I'm preconditioned to expect the worst. I hate it when *I* waste money, and I hate it when I'm attending to Medicaid folks who, by their zany ER visits, are doing nothing except wasting money. But—*and this is a big but*—on those rare occasions when a Medicaid recipient had a true emergency, I'd never begrudged giving them care. Same goes for the people who would never pay their hospital bills. (In fact, I'd sometimes give them whatever medicine they needed, if I had it at home.) Administrators, on the other hand, do begrudge such care. That's a sound business perspective, perhaps, but it's not very palatable from a humanitarian perspective. Now, do you want to be a customer, or a patient?

The next "customer," who I'll call Bob, was a retired GM worker whose wallet was stuffed with thousands of dollars. Turns out that he had a penchant for young women, but that's another story. In any event, he was the type of customer who could make an administrator salivate in gleeful anticipation. Naturally, he was the kind of folk we were expected to suck up to, but I was in no mood for sucking up. I'd seen Bob on numerous prior occasions, and I had always been put off by his personality.

---

[23]   I've never seen an administrator object to a psychiatric admission for a Medicaid patient, however. I suspect that was because their reimbursement schedules were better for psychiatric care than for other medical or surgical care.

Habitually, he never smiled. Instead, his countenance was perpetually contorted in a hateful scowl, and his diatribes were liberally peppered with profanity. I'm sure he was a big hit with the young ladies, with his engaging personality and scrawny physique.

At some point during his visit, Bob decided to move his truck, which was parked outside the emergency room. That's when the fun began. In the process of moving his vehicle, he managed to smash into two cars. After this demolition derby was over, he walked back into the ER as if nothing happened, and slipped back into his patient gown. One of the hospital security guards, who witnessed the collisions, dutifully informed me of the situation.

When I confronted Bob, his attitude was, *"So what?"* He was about as steady on his feet as would have been the equivalent mass of Jell-O®, and I was concerned that his driving would jeopardize him and anyone in his vicinity. He didn't see it that way, though. He was an excellent driver, he told me, and my concerns were without merit. He seemed shocked that I would have the temerity to question *him*, and when I suggested that he voluntarily surrender his driver's license, he went ballistic. Not to be dissuaded by a few dozen swear words and an angry spray of saliva, I called the police, who were equally impressed with his driving skills.

All in the name of protecting the public from this menace. Think of how pleased you'd be if I had let Mr. Coordination leave the ER in his truck, and he mowed over your 16-year-old sister. You would be mad, and justifiably so. Part of my job as an ER physician was to protect the public in such a manner, not just to kowtow to a well-heeled benefactor of the hospital. But did the administrators see it that way? Of course not! *He had money!* Who cares if he kills a few pedestrians on his way to the brothel? Don't make him mad, Pezzi, I was told—actually, threatened would be a more accurate description. I used to wonder if they taught morals in business school. Now I know.

■ "#^@$ you, you +>**@= S.O.B.!" What shocked me most was not this language, but the fact that it was emanating from the mouth of a two-year-old. His sentence structure was remarkably complex for someone that age, and his vocabulary of profane words was extensive. He made Bob, from the above story, seem like a charm school graduate. Parsing each sentence, I was struck that they were grammatically correct in spite of the fact that the majority of the words in them were vulgar. Sentence after sentence, paragraph after paragraph, the harangue went on, and on, and on.

"We have a little problem with his speech . . ." his mother meekly admitted. A *little* problem, I mused? This kid could make sailors blush! She continued, ". . . and we don't know where he picked up such language, either." I bet it wasn't from *Sesame Street.*

Given that this little tyke had been brought to the ER for his . . . uh, temper, I charted each and every precious phrase, thinking that it was important to capture his state of mind. In medical school, I was taught the importance of documenting such speech verbatim. The hospital brass didn't agree with that tenet, though. They felt I should have just said that the child was using "foul language." Somehow, that misses the mark. What does "foul language" mean? That the kid said, "Poo-poo"? Not quite. This child could concatenate a dozen obscene adjectives onto a number of sexually explicit verbs, producing epithets which could shock even Howard Stern. And I'm supposed to euphemize this by saying "foul language"? I don't think so. Ultimately, the primary function of medical documentation is to illustrate what is going on with a patient at a given time, so that later caregivers can be apprised of the patient's prior condition. Forming The Big Picture, you know.

The hospital bigwig's rationale for wanting me to tone down the documentation of the toddler's tirade was that it might offend someone, especially the kid's family. Yes, the child didn't swear, he "utilized disparaging language." His speech wasn't vile, it was "a reflection of his inner angst." Spare me the psycho-babble whitewashing, this youngster had enough inner rage to make Charles Manson seem like a pleasant dinner companion. Oh, but the child was covered by Blue Cross® insurance, meaning that he must always be depicted in a favorable light. Let us now bow to the Grand Pooh-Bah, the almighty dollar.

■ You might think that a patient who is requesting admission to a psychiatric ward would certainly be in need of help, right? After all, who else would desire such an admission? Who would? Given the right incentives, plenty of people would like to be admitted. Surprised? So was I.

Years ago, my conception of a mental hospital was a dank, dark, gloomy place in which remained leg irons and other vestiges of even more miserable times in the past. Orderlies, almost as warped as those they were treating, would chase after their subjects with syringes topped off with mind-bending drugs that would turn anyone into a zombie, if they weren't already. Fat-cat administrators, oblivious to the decadent commotion around them, would rarely venture from the confines of their plush offices . . .

Except for the bit about the administrators, I couldn't have been more wrong. Oh, I'm sure that Russian mental hospitals are not wallpapered with smiley faces, but American psychiatric wards have made great strides toward the eradication of their dungeon-like image. That's good, but it can be taken too far.

What's "too far"? A quiet, new, sparkling clean ward in which the patients would take day trips to a variety of local sites, play badminton on a rich green lawn sprinkled with picnic tables, engage in arts and crafts, watch television, go shopping, talk on the (free) phone, have pizza parties, read, and—even though it wasn't officially sanctioned—have sex. Day-passes were available to those whose wants could not be met by the hospital. *Is this a psychiatric ward, or Shangri-la?* The charges for the medicine, "rent," meals, and bedtime snacks are covered by the insurer. More often than not, the insurer is Medicaid, a.k.a., the taxpayers.

In my opinion, people who are truly mentally ill have less culpability for their problems than do people with most physical illnesses, and I certainly don't begrudge giving them care, even if I'm the one paying for it. However, most psychiatric admissions at these cushy hospitals are nothing more than shams, and the ultimate goal of the "patients" is not to get better, but to boink on a bed that *you're* paying for. After all, to them it's cheaper than Motel-6®.

Who would create a system so enjoyable that it could entice even those who were not mentally ill? Revenue-hungry hospital administrators, that's who. They know the word on the street will quickly spread that this is one bodaciously fun place to be, sort of a taxpayer-funded resort, more enjoyable than summer camp and without the need to sell boxes of candy to gain admission. Hence, the rooms will stay full, and the hospital coffers will be overflowing. The public outcry about $600 toilet seats is old news; where's the indignation about $600 pizza parties?

OK, next logical question. Why would ER physicians, in conjunction with psychiatrists, admit these people? Fear of a lawsuit, of course. In psychiatry, almost everything is subjective, and CYA tests to substantiate a diagnosis are unheard of. Consequently, hoards of would-be kooks and a mishmash of freeloaders pretend to be suicidal in order to be admitted. From their cohorts, they learn the magical words, tricks, and tantrums which seem to guarantee admission. Even when their acting skills are ludicrous and they are clearly *not* suicidal or even depressed, they're still routinely admitted. Why? The pseudo-psycho's secret weapon, the synthetic suicidal gesture. Let's say that Barbara has no more intention of killing herself than she does of ever getting a job and paying taxes, but the mean ER doctor and psychiatrist tell her to take a hike. This blows her plans of attending the Friday night pizza party, and the thought of missing out on the other perks is just too tempting. So, she will:

**a)** begin stomping her feet and storming from room to room in the ER, screaming that she is looking for a scalpel with which to commit suicide.

**b)** making sure that she is seen, drink from a container of Betadine®, which is generally sitting on the countertop in almost every room in the ER. Betadine® is not very toxic, but it makes for a good show.

**c)** sit down, and refuse to leave the hospital. She weighs about 260 pounds; would you like to eject her?

**d)** pull the keys from her purse, using one of them to scrape at her wrist as she screams, "*I'm . . . going . . . to . . . **die!***"

This is not a multiple choice question. Barbara (name changed to protect *blah, blah, blah*) really exists, and she has pulled all of these shenanigans in order to coerce me and the on-call psychiatrists to admit her on numerous occasions. Funny, in all the years of admitting her, if she were so suicidal, why did she never try it at home? Nonetheless, her reactive program of progressive escalation (*Patent Pending*) was carefully crafted to achieve the intended effect: admission.

Unfortunately, there are a lot of Barbaras out there, and they're draining billions of dollars from U.S. taxpayers. Think about that the next time you groan as your alarm clock awakens you at 6 a.m.—you're not going to work to support your wife and kids, you're going to work for Barbara. See, the predacious lawyers in this country are not just sticking their knives into the backs of doctors. They've got a knife in your back, too, and they're twisting it. They're the masters, and we're the slaves. Welcome to the New World Order.

If you're not already convinced that litigation has gotten out of hand, consider this: one lawyer made about as much money last year as was earned by *one thousand* pediatricians![24] Pediatricians are hardly paupers;

---

[24]    If you *still* don't think that litigation has gotten out of hand, consider this: recently, while giving a Sea-Doo® (a.k.a., "Jet Ski") ride to a 5-year-old, she sternly warned me, "*If anything happens to me while I'm on this thing, my parents will sue you!*" How rude! Referring to a Sea-Doo® as "this thing"! On to the next point. The fact that 5-year-old minds are already dwelling on lawsuits is alarming. Note, too, that she is automatically disavowing any personal culpability for such an injury; if she were injured, she presumes that it would be *my* fault. Typical finger-pointing. It's always the other guy . . .

Oddly, Little Miss Litigation uttered her threat while I was piloting the Sea-Doo® at an unconscionably reckless 3 m.p.h. At that speed, her greatest danger was dying from boredom.

imagine an income 1000 times greater—*it boggles the mind!* That's not respectable income, it's legalized extortion. And guess who is paying for it? You, your wife, your parents, your siblings, and your children. This attorney would like for you to believe that he's attacking *only* corporations. That's inane. Such costs are ultimately borne by someone, and the someone who ultimately provides money to corporations is you, the consumer. Increasing the risk and cost of doing business simply increases the cost of the goods and services provided by corporations.

The ever-present threat of malpractice litigation affects medical costs directly and indirectly, sending them on an alarming and increasingly costly upward spiral. Physicians know that they are essentially a legalized punching bag, made to bear the brunt of the responsibility for the collective shortcomings of science and society. Reflexively, physicians fight back with the only weapon at their disposal: CYA.

Let's return to the case of Barbara. Admitting her might cost $10,000. Would I admit her to stave off a lawsuit? *You bet I would!* I, and other doctors, have admitted her dozens—if not hundreds—of times. Granted, Barbara resides in one of the most litigious counties in a state that is known for its litigiousness, thus ensuring that Barbara and others of her ilk are thoroughly CYAed (since there are no CYA *tests*, we revert to a CYA *admission*). I have never met a physician who enjoyed the CYA game; to me, it is an abomination, albeit a necessary one.

If Barbara were truly suicidal, yeah, sure, let's admit her. Some people may question spending $10,000 on an adult whose only conception of work is cashing welfare checks (having been as successful milking the welfare system as she is in coercing physicians), but society does not permit physicians to place a monetary value upon life. So, Barb is admitted, again, and again, and again. In total, she's drained over a million dollars from the taxpayers in twenty-some years of life. What has she contributed in return? Absolutely nothing; she has *never* had a job. I feel sorry for those who cannot work, but I loathe those who refuse to work. Barbara fits the latter category. She is not a moron. She is not crippled. She's definitely odd, but she does not meet the medical criteria of insanity. A few decades ago, her shenanigans would have bought her a one-way ticket to a dingy state mental hospital. However, society has decreed that these borderline fruitcakes should roam free. And that they do. Many of them quickly figure out that their path of least resistance through life is to make a career out of sponging off a society that is, by its overgenerosity, making it a viable option to be a lifelong leech.

*Journal of dubious*

# EMERGENCY CARE

**EXAMINING THE TENUOUS NECESSITY OF CATERING TO NON-EMERGENCIES**   **May 1998**

*Acting-out vs. just plain acting: the Oscars for the best ER performances of all time.*

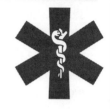

*Motel-6®or the ER:* the results of our exclusive popularity poll.

*Best bet for a bedtime snack:* a fast-food restaurant? Nope, they'll make you pay. Go to the ER—it won't be fast, and it may not be food . . . but it's FREE! It's the American way!

## A JDEC Exclusive:

Bizarre reasons
for dialing

# 911

*Can't get a date on Saturday night?* Go to the ER! If there's a more legitimate emergency, we can't think of it!

*Looking for a reason to go to the ER?* Look no further! JDEC previews the renovations of six popular emergency rooms. The Parade of Homes is over, but the ERs are always open! A surefire crowd-pleaser!

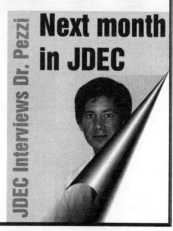

**Next month in JDEC**

JDEC Interviews Dr. Pezzi

Having far more common sense and far less money, other societies refuse to kowtow to such people. Are there hordes of oddballs committing suicide in these countries? Of course not. Their oddballs know that wacky behavior will get them nowhere. So, they don't do it; in the process of adapting to this realization, they become less odd. This impetus for normalization is sadly lacking in American society today. Whatever your foible or shortcoming, it can be blamed on someone else. But there is a price to be paid for this diversion of responsibility. It weakens the individual, and society. Permissive, undemanding, "anything goes," set-no-standards parents raise children who grow up to be wild, if not monsters. Increasingly, American society is assuming the parental role—and frankly, it's flubbing it.

■ Believe it or not, but emergency rooms are an integral link in the seedy world of narcotic abuse. Every ER in the nation is frequently besieged by a never-ending stream of clowns who pretend to be in agony in an attempt to bamboozle the ER doc into giving them narcotics, which they then use for their own enjoyment, or for sale. This latter activity can be quite lucrative. Since prescription narcotics are highly prized on the street for their purity and potency, they command top dollar. Working part-time, entrepreneurs who specialize in such narcotic diversion can easily make more money than the doctors they're hoodwinking. Fortunately, most ER doctors are ethically disgusted by such junkies, and make it a point of pride to ferret out these impostors.

Some of the tactics used by these fakes are ludicrously transparent. They may claim to be on vacation, and state that they forgot to bring their drugs with them. Stopping by the ER "just for a refill," they attempt to sway the physician with such powerful logic as, "Well, my doctor gives it to me!" Sorry to disappoint them, but physicians are not prescription-writing robots who perform upon command. Other patients claim to have lost a prescription for a narcotic, and request a replacement. Funny, but I've *never* seen a patient lose a prescription for an antibiotic. Hmmmmm . . . Others, schooled in the latest techniques of armchair psychologists, will feign unfamiliarity with the desired narcotic, stammering or otherwise mispronouncing it as their eyes betray the zeal of their opiate longing. "Uh, uh, I think it's Per-Per-Perco-Percodan®, or something." *Right*. It's odd that patients never have such difficulty with the pronunciation of Motrin® or Toradol®.

People who are suffused with the "have it your way" mentality typically respond with self-righteous indignation when their request for a specific narcotic is not granted immediately. They act as if they're able to select the desired drug from a menu, expecting the physician to accede graciously, just as they are accommodated when they walk into McDonald's® or Burger King®. "I want some Demerol®, and I don't want any of that generic stuff, either!" Extra mayo, hold the lettuce, and a slice of cheese, too? Happy to serve you, master. Right away, master. Unfortunately for them, the DEA (Drug Enforcement Agency) does not permit physicians to hand out narcotics as if they were M&M's®. Isn't life tough?

■ Some patients favor a less heavy-handed approach in the procurement of narcotics. While I appreciate their gracious consideration of my feelings (after all, who likes to be bossed around?), I still refuse if there is anything fishy about their supposed need for a narcotic. Others dispense with any pretense of legitimacy, and get right down to business. Monkey business. That was Jenny's specialty.

"You're a doctor, right?" Given that I was the only physician working in the ER at that time, I knew this question had been posed merely for rhetorical effect. "So," she continued, "if you're a doctor, that means you can prescribe drugs, right?"

Another obviously rhetorical question, but I decided to answer anyway. "Yes, I can."

"I'd like some morphine tablets," she said.

"Why do you want morphine?"

"To sell it. I'll pay you $5 a pill. A hundred pills is $500."

I could do the math myself. She didn't know that I'd once beaten Bill Gates in a math test. "I don't sell drugs for money."

Jenny was not easily dissuaded. "But think of the money you could make! You wouldn't have to work here anymore."

Now *that* was tempting! Kidding aside . . . "If I had wanted to be a drug pusher, I wouldn't have bothered to go through college, medical school, and residency. I am *not* going to sell prescriptions."

"Well, would you do it if I sleep with you?"

"Uh . . ."

She smiled, thinking she was getting somewhere.

For the sake of the nation, it's a good thing that such an offer had not been made to President Clinton in exchange for selling nuclear technology to the Red Chinese. "Uh, no. I have a girlfriend." That, and I have a fear of federal prison, or wherever they put wayward doctors.

"So? I'm not going to tell your girlfriend."

Jenny was missing the point. The high-octane life in the criminal underworld was not appealing to me. "I wouldn't do it even if I didn't have a girlfriend."

She seemed a bit crestfallen. "Aren't you attracted to me?"

"That's not the issue," I answered. This was the only semi-cryptic answer I could think of at the time.

"I used to be a model. Most guys think I'm really pretty. They're always asking me out, and trying to get me in bed. You wouldn't believe some of the things they try."

"Perhaps they should offer you morphine tablets," I suggested.

"Ha, ha, very funny, Doctor." With that, she gave me a quick smirk, and then stood up from the stretcher upon which she had been sitting. I thought she was going to leave, but she wasn't ready to call it a day just yet. It was time to employ the ultimate female weapon: tears.

"Oh, Doctor, you don't know . . . you don't know how hard I've had it. I'm just . . . (more sobbing) . . . just trying to make a living. I don't use the drugs, either. I bet you thought I did, though. No, I just sell them. Just sell them . . . (more crying and a few self-righteous snorts) . . . but I only sell to good people. No junkies, no criminals, nobody who'd hurt anybody. They just want a nice pleasant buzz. What's the harm in that? Can't you help me out?"

"Sure I can," I responded.

"You can?" She seemed surprised, and a look of relief and joy spread over her face. She took a couple of steps, and threw her arms around me.

"Yes. I can use some help working in my yard this weekend. I'll pay you $12 an hour," I offered. End of hug.

She seemed piqued, as if I'd asked her to do something unspeakably degrading and demeaning. "You want *me* to *work* . . . in your *yard*?"

"What's wrong with that? It's how I paid my way through college and medical school."

"Forget it! I thought you wanted to help me! What do you think I am, a slave?"

# *I'm not* that *gullible*

■ Some people expect that ER doctors will believe *anything* you tell them. Not quite. While non-ER physicians might find this hard to believe (or, they may simply be unaware of the statistics), gaining acceptance to an ER residency program is *the* most competitive venture in postgraduate medical education. Think it's difficult getting into a residency for orthopedic surgery or neurosurgery? It's a piece of cake compared to getting into an ER program. Having worked for years as an ER doctor, I have to wonder about the intelligence of anyone who actually wants to ~~abuse themselves~~ —I mean, be an ER doc. Kidding aside, ER doctors are anything but stupid. Mary didn't believe that, though. Want to hear a wild story? Good.

Joe went over to Jim's home. Jim, a friend of Joe, was making love to his girlfriend, Mary. Without being too graphic, Jim couldn't satisfy Mary, so he got up and left the home. But not Joe. He decided to give it the old college try, seeing if he could satisfy Mary. Joe and Mary were thoroughly enjoying themselves when Jim returned. Jim asked Joe to get off his girlfriend. Joe had something else on his mind, however, and continued on his merry way. Jim then tried pulling Joe off. No go. Jim then got his pistol and shot Joe in the back of the head. What a way to end a friendship, eh?

The paramedics brought what was left of Joe into the ER. He never had a chance. After I determined that his brain injury was incompatible with life, I put on my detective's cap and began sleuthing. Mary claimed that after Joe had finished making love (well, having sex is a more apt description), he got Jim's gun and shot himself. Oh, I believe *that!* I've thought of many things after intercourse, but somehow suicide has never crossed my mind. Furthermore, Joe was shot in the *back* of the head. The angle of the wound indicated that it was not self-inflicted. Besides, who shoots themselves in the back of the head? Having precious little common sense and no appreciation of forensic science, Mary actually thought we would fall for the story that she and Jim had concocted. Guess again.

■ People who are shot or stabbed by someone they know are often unwilling to divulge the name of their assailant. Their reluctance is often rooted in the fact that the shoot*ee* is just as much of a criminal as the shoot*er*, and the shoot*ee* would like to keep this a secret. Consequently, these erudite scholars oftentimes concoct a lame explanation, most of which seem to follow a script: "I was just mindin' my own business, and then he walks up and shoots me!"

Perhaps. Some innocent people are shot, but that usually happens to churchgoing grandmothers and people who are carjacked on their way to a PTA meeting. It's usually easy for the ER doctor to differentiate these people from those who are seedy. Seedy people seem to be constitutionally unable to devise plausible stories, but they try anyway. They may as well hang a sign around their neck which says:

**Ladies and gentlemen, the story you are about to hear is patent bullshit. The details have been changed in a pathetic attempt to protect the guilty.**

The only thing missing is the music from the old TV show *Dragnet.*

I've heard even worse, but Ernie's story is typical. "Well, Doc, I don't know who shot me." He went on to claim that he was shot in a city about 170 miles south, and he hitchhiked a ride on the freeway to come to this ER. Hmmm . . . I didn't know that people felt comfortable about letting blood-soaked strangers enter their cars. Furthermore, I couldn't imagine driving 170 miles to find an emergency room. I used to work in the city in which he said he was shot, and I knew there were four major ER's in that city. So I inquired as to why he didn't go to one of those facilities. "I don't like them. They don't have good reputations."

That was news to me. Situated in the Murder Capital of the World (no joke, unfortunately), they had plenty of experience dealing with such cases. I then asked, "Why did you come up here?"

"Oh, because this hospital has a much better reputation!"

Now I knew he was lying. "This" hospital has about as much experience with gunshot wounds as Michael Jackson does with adult women. My face must have appeared disbelieving, as if to say, "Surely you jest, you fool."

"Oh, no," he said as he continued to dig himself deeper, "I've heard that this is the place to come if you have a gunshot wound!"

Thinking to myself, "Why, because my colleagues have a reputation for being gullible?" I'd heard enough, and left to call the police. Sure enough, he'd been shot around here—he was just trying to keep the true story from coming out. Better luck next time, bub.

■"What do you think it is, Doctor?" Gary held the bottle of Mt. Dew® up to the light, and gently sloshed the remaining contents. He said that he noticed something in the bottle while drinking from it, and shortly thereafter became nauseated.

"I don't know," I replied.

Gary continued, "I think it's a condom."

"A *condom*?" I asked.

"Yes, a condom. A *used* condom."

Hmmm . . . such a conjecture requires a vivid imagination, or poor eyesight. Or greed. Gary was ranting on and on about how he was going to sue the bottling company.

"What makes you think it's a used condom?" I inquired.

"You see them little globs floating around in the pop?"

"Yes," I answered.

"It's sperm," he opined.

Short of finding a fragment of rubber tattooed with "Trojan®" or "Ramses®," I wouldn't know how to conclusively demonstrate whether the debris in the bottle was a fragmented condom. But sperm? I'm a medical doctor. That's something I could determine. I took a sample of the soft drink, and examined it under a microscope. No sperm. Had there been sperm, I suppose it would have given new meaning to the term "Mt. Dew."

Informed of the absence of sperm, Gary seemed disappointed, and increasingly irate. "I know it's sperm!" he shouted. With this proclamation he drew the attention of several people in the ER. He pointed to the bottle, and raised it to the light once more. "That's a condom in there. I know it is! Can't you see it?"

I saw some amorphous globs floating in the bottle, but I doubted that Mt. Dew® would produce such a transformation of latex. "I see something in the bottle," I replied, "but it doesn't remind me of a condom."

"You're stupid, Doctor! You can't even tell a condom when it's right in front of you!"

Gary's addled cousin, who accompanied him to the ER, could not resist chiming in. "I know it's a condom, too. I saw him put it in. But he didn't put no sperm in there. He ain't no pree-vert, ya know."

■ One of the most common ways in which drug addicts attempt to trick ER physicians into giving them narcotics is by pretending to have a kidney stone. Some people are good actors, and know of several ways to present a convincing case. Others, however, have no idea of what they're doing, and they make some rather comical errors.

Such as Marty. From the get-go, my gut instinct told me that he was a fake, but he claimed to be in utter agony. I requested a urine specimen from him, as I would often do if I wasn't convinced that a patient really had a stone. "If I have a stone, will you give me a shot for pain?" he begged.

"Sure I will. No problem."

"Thanks, Doc, 'cause this pain is really bad. I've never had anything like it before."

"I'm sure you haven't," I said.

As he walked out of the restroom a minute later, he handed me the specimen cup. In it was urine—and a stone.

"See, Doc, I passed a kidney stone. It's right in here." He pointed it out, as if I couldn't see it for myself. He seemed pleased.

I was not. "That's a stone, alright, but it's not a *kidney* stone."

I knew that he knew, but he was hoping that I didn't know. "W-w-w-what do you think it is?" he stammered.

"Looks like granite to me," I answered. The rock was jagged, and about half an inch in diameter. If he had passed such a stone (which was virtually impossible), his urine would have looked like blood, but it was a nice bright yellow. Kidney stones that are spontaneously passed, on the other hand, are typically 1/8" in diameter, or smaller, and they're usually associated with blood in the urine.

"No, Doc, really, I passed that stone, and I know that I have more inside me, 'cause I'm still in pain!"

Didn't he know the jig is up, I thought? "You may have some rocks in you, but they're not in your urinary system."

He feigned concern. "Uh, uh, where could they be?"

I tapped my index finger twice on the side of my head, and walked away.

# The final egress

■ After a patient dies, it's not uncommon for family members to ask the physician if their departed relative suffered just before death. When I was working in the ER, it didn't take me long to realize that they want to hear there had been no suffering. Even though I'm adamantly opposed to lying, I think this is clearly a special case in which it's better to lie than to unnecessarily add to the suffering of the surviving relatives. What possible good could result from admitting that their death had, indeed, been agonizing? On occasion, when I thought it was obvious—even to a layperson—that the patient suffered, and that no one would believe me if I said otherwise, I'd concoct a story to make it seem plausible that the suffering had been slight.

Before deciding to discuss this topic, I debated the merits of its inclusion. While not wanting to undermine the comforting buffer of well-intended deception, I'm concerned that continuing to ignore this topic will only perpetuate practices which make such suffering unavoidable.

When death is imminent and the terminal patient has previously been declared "no code," it is often appropriate and ethical to administer a drug (such as morphine) that substantially eases pain and the fear of death. Oftentimes, however, this isn't done. Why? Well, there are a few major stumbling blocks which either botch, or outright preclude, the implementation of this tactic.

• Frequently, patients are rushed to an emergency room at the last minute. To begin with, a pell-mell journey to the ER in an ambulance with sirens blaring is not an ideal way to begin one's worldly egress. This is generally a reaction to a lack of planning, or a lack of time imposed by a precipitous decline. If time permits, hospice care is certainly preferable. As a rule, ambulance personnel will not make the decision that the patient's proximity to death, and overall prognosis, is sufficient to warrant the administration of a drug that eases—but often hastens—death.

• Assuming the patient does make it to the ER alive, there is still no guarantee that the amelioration of the agony of death will take precedence over the attempted prevention of death. Doctors are often reluctant to "kill" people, even when the choice is giving a patient three minutes of bliss, or five minutes of sheer torture. Notwithstanding the efforts of Dr. Kevorkian, physicians are still afraid of being sued, or even being charged with murder. If you accompany a dying family member to the ER in such a circumstance, immediately inform the doctor of the patient's and family's acceptance of the impending death, and stress that the relief of suffering is paramount. Doctors are cognizant of the fact that there are more than a few people still harboring the delusion that every death is a surefire indication of malpractice, so they are understandably unnerved at the prospect of expediting death, even when it's the only humane option.

• Acting on their own convictions, nurses may refuse to administer morphine (or a similarly-intended drug), or even to allow the physician to do so. In hospitals, nurses hold the keys—literally—to the narcotic box. If they refuse to open the box, or to relinquish the keys, the dying patient will not receive the drug. Shortly after becoming a physician, I was involved in such a case. An elderly man was dying of lung cancer, and he was clearly in distress, gasping for breath and drowning in his own secretions. He, his family, his doctor, and his oncologist (cancer specialist) had previously agreed on a "no code" status, and he was brought to the hospital merely to ease his suffering. This seemed entirely reasonable to me, so I asked the nurse to administer morphine. She refused this order, and—with hands on her hips—she let it be known that she wouldn't give me the keys to the narcotic box, either. She explained that her religious convictions prevented her from even indirectly participating in a death, even in such an extenuating circumstance. I thought it was rather arrogant for her to place *her* religious convictions above those of the patient, his family, the decisions of the patient's doctors, and simple humanity.

■ We tried to save her life. Though we were reluctant to admit defeat, we had to stop the code. She wasn't going to make it. She was dead. And she was only 21.

Like many fire victims, Becky died not of heat per se but of smoke inhalation. She was living with other addicts in a dope house. In the middle of the night, someone had boarded up the windows and doors from the outside, and then tossed in a Molotov cocktail. The house was quickly engulfed by fire and smoke, with its horrified victims trapped inside.

After the code was over, we searched her body for identification. In searching for that, we found something else: a letter she'd just written to her parents. In it, she expressed sorrow for the pain she knew she had caused them, and for the time that she had wasted. But things would be different now. She was giving up drugs, and she hoped to find a job to pay for college. She said that she was leaving the next morning to spend a few weeks with an old high school friend who had moved to Maine. After that, she'd be home in time for Christmas.

I contemplated what to do with that letter. Should I forward it to her parents, who might rejoice in their daughter's eager plans for a fresh start in life? Or would the letter only cause more pain to her parents, forever haunting them with the knowledge that she had *almost* just made it. It didn't take me long to decide. I threw the letter in a trash can, and walked out of the room.

■ Time for a trivia break. Nitroglycerin paste is applied to the chest wall of some heart patients. If a patient bearing nitro paste requires CPR and is shocked, the nitro can actually explode. The first time I witnessed this I was more than a bit surprised, but it was all there: the ka-boom, the flash, the burnt gunpowder smell—or was that the smell of burnt flesh? I shouldn't have been surprised, though. After all, it *is* nitroglycerin, and the electrical energy of the shock is sufficient to detonate the nitro.

■ As an emergency physician, I've seen some gruesome things: disemboweled patients, mangled bones sticking through skin, splattered brains, heads torn from the neck, and amputations of all sorts. I've seen people scalped and intentionally splashed with acid (yes, it's the same old story: Girl A perceives that Girl B is much prettier; Girl A dumps acid onto Girl B to eliminate B's competitive advantage). I've seen people shot by all types of guns; close-range shotgun blasts and high-power rifle wounds are by far the worst. (Incidentally, Clint Eastwood is a much better actor than he is a ballistician: in one of the Dirty Harry movies, he claims that a .44 Magnum "will blow your head clean off." That's just Hollywood hyperbole.) I've also seen people "shot" by carpentry nailers, and objects thrown from lawnmower blades. I've seen people run over by cars, trucks, buses, tractors, motorcycles, ATV's, boats, and snowmobiles. I've also seen two men run over by their wives; one with a golf cart, and one with a riding lawnmower. Both were unintentional—just typical woman drivers, I suppose.

The most grisly sight? In the evening, Wanda had been strolling down a sidewalk with her infant when she was confronted by a rapist. Witnesses said that she told him to #μ¢! himself, which enraged the scumbag. He stabbed her neck repeatedly with a foot-long kitchen knife, penetrating from side to side. When Wanda came into the ER—stone dead, of course—the knife was still skewered through her neck, but its handle had been torn off by the last violent thrust. Wanda's face seemed to be contorted in pain. Not surprisingly.

This last case illustrates the type of violence which I found particularly senseless. The scenario is generally this: the criminal approaches the victim, and demands something (sex, designer tennis shoes, a leather jacket, or a cool T-shirt). The victim refuses, and is murdered. The irony is that the criminal never got what he sought. After all, who wants a blood-soaked pair of sneakers?

■ The paramedics brought an assault victim with a cardiac arrest to the ER. His head was wrapped with several layers of gauze. Shortly after his arrival in the ER, as we continued the resuscitative efforts, I decided to see what was under the gauze. I removed it, and announced that the code was over. There was no point in continuing it—his skull was shattered, and chunks of brain tissue were falling out.

■ On another occasion, I was undressing a man who had been brought to the ER in a coma, searching for a clue which might explain his problem. As I removed his socks, the skin of his feet peeled off along with the socks—they had literally grown together, and both were rotten. The smell was nauseating. I deemed this the *toxic sock syndrome.*

■ The 911 call came in as "difficulty breathing." It wasn't asthma, it wasn't pneumonia, it wasn't an allergic reaction, and it wasn't heart failure. On second thought, it was *sort of* heart failure—but not of the patient.

Michelle was a rather diminutive member of the world's oldest profession. One day, while at work, one of her customers collapsed on her. Not unconscious. Dead. His heart had stopped. Unfortunately for Michelle, her customer was a corpulent 400-plus-pounder. Displacing 400+ pounds of Jell-O proved to be an insurmountable task for a heroin-ravaged body. She screamed for help, but no one came running to help this damsel in distress. Within minutes, she was exhausted from the effort of breathing with so much weight on her. She thought that her life was over. Such an ignominious end!

Then she saw it. The telephone! Taxpayer-supported 911! She was able to reach the phone on the table next to the bed, and she dialed those magic numbers. Help would be there within minutes. She was saved.

Had she not been saved, I wouldn't have had the opportunity to see her when she came into the ER a week later with both gonorrhea and herpes. She wasn't in a good mood. "Man, I've been f-----!"

That characterization seemed apropos. I thought about it for a moment, and then responded, "Yes, you have."

■ During my ER residency, one of the many requirements was to spend a couple of days riding with the paramedics in their ambulances. That was a real eye-opening experience. The intended goal was to gain some firsthand knowledge of pre-hospital care, but there were other lessons to be learned as well. What I found particularly striking was the filth in most of the homes we visited. Hundreds of dirty dishes covered the countertops, each encrusted with moldy, decaying bits of food. The floors were similarly covered with chunks of food, animal waste, newspapers, clothes, and all sorts of junk. Walking across a room often required that I clear a path by pushing things out of my way. Flies were buzzing everywhere, and the odors were simply repugnant. Some of the homes had bars on their windows, which seemed to me to be an unnecessary deterrent.

One of the homes was occupied by a LOL with SDC—a little old lady with several dozen cats. The cats that I'd known as a child were fastidiously clean. However, when cats are deprived of the opportunity to use a litter box or to go outside, they devise some rather creative means of relieving themselves. Such as in an open container of flour. Glancing at this, a couple of marks indicated that the LOL had scooped some flour from the container after the cats had last used it. She was baking cookies for the church bake sale, she said.

I also discovered that there was some correlation between filth and inattention to medical care. Some folks come to the ER after literally one sneeze, and others don't bother to call for an ambulance until a day after a family member stopped breathing.

"Clarence there, he laid down on the couch after supper last night. Said he had some indigestion. He didn't complain of nothin' today, though, but he never said nothin' today, either. You think he's dead?"

I checked for a pulse. No pulse. His skin was cool. He'd obviously been dead for several hours. When I used my stethoscope to listen for heart or lung sounds, I saw a cockroach scurry from his gaping mouth. Startled, I jumped back. "Yes, he's dead."

■ Jackie was walking to a local convenience store to buy some snacks and to rent a video. On her way, a fellow teenager that she knew from the neighborhood stopped his car and asked if she wanted a ride. Sure, why not? She hopped in.

She never made it to the store. Instead, Andy took her to a deserted flophouse, where he raped her several times over a period of three hours. If she told anyone, he threatened, he'd do the same to her little sister.

In the ER, Jackie was hysterical. Jackie's brother, Frank, was ballistic. "I'll kill that S.O.B.!"

Frank wasn't just blowing off steam, I later found out. A few days later, Andy—whose name I recognized—came into the ER, D.O.A.

One of the nurses mused, "Who could have done this?"

"I haven't got a clue," I responded.

■ When I was an ER resident years ago, I was working one particularly bloody weekend in which a record was set for the most murders in that city in any weekend period in its history. I can't recall the exact number of murders, but it was something like 52. The major newspaper in that metro area ran a story about this murder spree, synopsizing the case of each of the victims. One problem, though. They'd missed a few. While reading the article, I thought of the patients I'd had who were murdered, but were not mentioned in the article. What about Ronnie? And what about Aaron? And what about Bobbie? Clearly, no one could keep up with the carnage—not even the newspaper.

■ I'd just explained to Tina that her husband didn't make it. He had been electrocuted at work when he was working on a circuit breaker box while standing in a puddle of water—not a real bright thing to do, by the way. Tina didn't seem particularly upset, though. I attributed this to her being in a state of shock (no pun intended). Little did I know that it was *I* who would soon be in a state of shock.

Matter-of-factly, Tina expressed her final wish for her husband: she wanted me to "harvest" his penis, and give it to her! "It's the only thing about him that I really liked, anyway."

# Miscellaneous ramblings

■ You think *I'm* blunt?  In comparison to some of my colleagues, I'm the epitome of decorum.  Some of their comments have left me—*even me*—reeling in disbelief that they'd have the temerity to say such a thing.  For instance . . .

It was around shift-change time.  I was coming on duty for the night shift, and Jill, the ER physician who'd worked the preceding shift, was preparing to leave.  We were standing in the nursing station, discussing who-knows-what, when an *elderly* lady was wheeled into the ER on an ambulance stretcher.  She was about 100 years old, but didn't look it.  She looked 200, if that were possible.  I've seen my share of centenarians, and I've never suffered from the delusion that 100 years of life didn't excuse a whole lot of wrinkles, sags, and bags.  Still, when I saw her, I was shocked.  Shocked that she was still alive.  Shocked that I'd soon be faced with the task of extending a life that seemed to be already overextended.  But I was mute.  Typically, Jill was not.  "She's a f-----g *fossil*!  What the hell does she want us to do?  *Save* her?  She should have been dead when Eisenhower was President!"

And then there is Jack.  Jack is a nurse whose behavior and speech would ordinarily warrant a depiction of its being in a class by itself, except that I've met several others who were equally outspoken.  What triggered this latest outburst was an ER patient named Linda who, unfortunately, complained of pelvic pain.  Unfortunate for me, since this necessitated doing a pelvic exam.

Contrary to popular notion, virtually all sane doctors do not relish such exams.  Doctors who are looking for titillation at work are looking for trouble.  Even when *my* sex life seemed perpetually on hold, I'd never get a vicarious thrill from doing a pelvic exam.  Well, I lie.  Maybe once or twice—hey, I'm human, and they were incredibly gorgeous.  But not Linda, who could spin a dial on a bathroom scale past the zero mark twice, and who sported more fur on her forearms than did most lumberjacks.  Then it hit me.  No, not some brilliant genetic diagnosis to explain her appearance.  What hit me was the stench of rotting yeast.  Not a vaginal yeast infection, but what's termed candidal inframammary and infrapannicular intertrigo.  Let's not get hung up on big words—it's just a yeast infection of the skin in the folds beneath the breasts and the apron of fat hanging over her lower belly.  If you've never encountered such a thing, count yourself among the lucky. To put it succinctly, it's gross. It's also a slimy, pasty oozing of yeasty pus, which justifies the former characterization. Having been trained in Detroit, where soap is apparently a four-letter word, I'd seen it before, and my dinner was in no immediate danger of retrograde expulsion. Poor Jack was spared the sight of the fetid fungal intertrigo, but who could ignore her teeth? Or, more precisely, what was left of them. Stumps, black stumps, coated with the requisite pus. A few spindly teeth remained, and one—loose in its socket—nauseatingly flapped back and forth when she spoke. Not surprisingly, her breath was a tad less appealing than that of a bear who'd just polished off a mound of sun-ripened carrion. Then she dropped the bombshell, mentioning that she'd had a baby a few months ago. Jack's face contorted in disbelief, and he darted out of the room. I followed. "Who on Earth could go to bed with *that?*" he asked rhetorically. "She's a *Neanderthal!* She's *disgusting!* There isn't enough booze in the world to get me drunk enough to sleep with her! How could *anybody* do it?" Except for postulating a similarly endowed male, I was equally stumped.

Back to the pelvic exam. I entered the room with more than my usual level of trepidation, and three layers of gloves. I *thought* I was adequately protected. In most circumstances, I would have been, but not with Linda. During the procedure she clamped her thighs together, and I was sandwiched in between. Disconcertingly, this almost made me fall forward, onto the intertrigo slime. Quicksand would have been a kinder fate. "Let me go!" I implored. She squeezed harder, and I began losing my balance, and my patience. Deciding that the time had come to set aside physician propriety, my instinct for self-preservation took over. Using all of my strength, I spread my upper arms, which released the pincer grip of her gelatinous thighs, allowing me to free myself. Stepping back, I was sweating, but yeast-free.

▪ A bit more graphic story that the squeamish are advised to skip.

My Intro to Intertrigo course was provided by a 660-pound woman who was admitted through the ER in the summertime when I was a third-year med student doing my rotation (i.e., course) in medicine. Her apartment had no air conditioning and she hadn't bathed in months. Coupled with her obesity, she was a prime candidate for intertrigo. And what a terrible case of it she had! Beneath her massive breasts (I have no idea how to quantitate their size, but they must have been several gallons each) was a fetid patch of red skin oozing a thick, slimy layer of yeast. A similar patch was present beneath the rolls of fat on her lower abdomen, and around her vulva. I discovered the latter when I attempted to perform a pelvic examination (complete examinations were required for that rotation). Much to my utter embarrassment, I was unable to locate the opening to her vagina. I knew where it was *supposed* to be, of course, but when I inserted the vaginal speculum and opened its blades, I could see nothing but fat—and gobs of yeasty slime. I tried a few more times, but I still couldn't locate her vagina.

Reluctant to admit my failure, I approached one of the residents on my service. He said that he would help me. Much to my horror, he donned a short pair of gloves (which didn't extend beyond his wrists), and walked into the patient's room. In his pleasingly accented voice, he proclaimed, "Don't worry, I find it!" Stepping back from the patient, he then literally dove forward with his outstretched right arm firmly grasping the speculum. Penetrating through a good eight inches of fat, he'd indeed located the vagina and, in one fell swoop, inserted the speculum inside it. "There it is!" he proudly exclaimed. Seeing that several inches of his bare forearm skin were in contact with the slime, a sudden wave of nausea overcame me.

■ Another gross story. We called her Maggie. You'll soon know why.

One of the many hazards of injecting street drugs is that they're often contaminated with germs. Some of these germs filter out of the bloodstream and cause festering sores. This rotting meat attracts flies, and flies lay eggs, which develop into maggots. With a bit of attention to personal cleanliness, it would be possible to abort the life cycle of the flies, but junkies are not known for their attention to hygiene.

Bonnie was a junkie who had been admitted to the hospital on a number of occasions for drug-related complications. This time, she had a large, oozing sore behind one of her knees. Swimming in the sore's slime layer were a number of maggots—hence the "Maggie" nickname. What surprised me more than the presence of the maggots was the fact that Maggie seemed totally oblivious to their presence. Even when we told her about the maggots, she gave us a "so what?" shrug and went back to reading her *National Enquirer*. I thought that inquiring minds wanted to know, but I was wrong.

■ Training in Detroit, I was taught to use the lingo of the locals, instead of what I thought were universally understood terms. For example, I'd never have guessed that asking a patient, "Have you ever had surgery?" would often elicit a negative response even though the patient had undergone multiple prior surgeries. Instead, we were taught to phrase the question in what I thought was a relatively crude manner, asking "Anybody ever cut on you?" *What* has happened to the English language? Is "surgery" really such an esoteric word?

This linguistic chasm was certainly unfortunate, but it did provide for some entertaining moments of locker room humor. The case of the new mother comes to mind.

Betty had just given birth to a daughter, and she was discussing the choice of a name with her roommate, who was equally clueless. Mulling over the possibilities, Betty considered a word that she'd recently heard on the obstetric ward. "Vagina, that be a nice name . . . hmm, I think I'll call her 'Vagina'." Admittedly a euphonious word, the two women agreed that "Vagina" would indeed be a nice name for a girl.

When the time came to relay the name choice to one of the hospital's personnel, the shocked worker exclaimed, "Uh, you can't name her 'Vagina'!" To which the Mom replied, "I be her Mother, and I can name her whatever I wants to!" This prompted the worker to explain just what a vagina was, but the Mom was skeptical. "That ain't a *vagina*—it's a *cootchie!*"

■ "I'm sorry that you lost your home." I was trying to be sympathetic with a homeless man, Fred.

"Why should *you* be sorry?" he asked. "Heck, *I'm* not sorry."

This surprised me. "You're not?"

"Not a bit. I used to have a home in the suburbs, a wife, three kids, and a job at Ford Motor. One day I woke up and said, 'I've had enough of this shit.' So I walked out. Don't regret it a bit, either."

This didn't exactly mesh with what I'd heard from the politically correct crowd. Implicit in their "Help The Homeless" slogan was the notion that the homeless wanted help. That made sense to me, but not to Fred.

"But you don't have to live on the streets," I implored. "You have a home and a family . . ."

"Yes, I did. But I gave it all up. I much prefer this life."

"You do?" I asked incredulously.

"You bet I do!"

In disbelief, I asked, "How could you?"

"What's this country all about?"

"Opportunity?"

"Not *opportunity*," he declared, "it's *freedom*. Before, my life was ruled by a damned clock. Get up at a certain time. Be to work by a certain time. Get so much work done within a certain time. Be home by a certain time. After a while, I felt like I was a dang robot. And then there were the bills. I had a lot of money, but I also had a lot of bills. The mortgage, the car, the insurance, the utilities, the food, the taxes—no matter how much money you make, there's always someone to take it from you. Is this freedom? Hell, no! Freedom is doing what you want to do. Before, I was doing what everyone else wanted me to do. Just like a robot. Now I do what *I* want to do. I get up when I want. I do whatever I want all day long. No bills, no clocks, no nagging, no threats. Now that's freedom. There's a lot to be said for it."

He had a point.

▪ One of my most embarrassing moments in medicine occurred years ago when I was on-call for plastic surgery. After I arrived home from the hospital, I drank a beer. This was a rare thing for me, as I'm ordinarily not much of a drinker. As luck would have it, though, I'd no sooner set the beer can down when my beeper went off. Oh s---!, I'd forgotten that I was on-call. It was a message to call the ER. Yikes, what do I do now?

There was no escape, so I called the ER. They had a patient who had his right hand severely chewed up after he inserted it into his mower deck, while the mower was running. So much for Darwin's theory of evolution, I thought.

Well, there was no getting out of this one. I had to go to the ER, beer breath or not. This seemed to be an unseemly breach of professionalism, and I was feeling the brunt of whatever compunction my brain could dish out. I was also afraid that someone would smell the alcohol on my breath, and that I'd have the medical Gestapo after me.

But I lucked out, plain and simple. The patient was so plastered that he saturated all of the air within a thirty foot radius with the smell of booze. Eureka! A light went off in my head—I'll just stick close to the patient, and everyone will assume that *he* was the source of the alcohol. Whenever I needed something which wasn't in the immediate area, I just asked someone to get it for me. They were eager to oblige, probably because they wanted the patient discharged from the ER, and that wouldn't happen until I was finished with the surgery. Knowing my sensitivity to alcohol, I took my time, making sure that everything was perfect as I repaired his numerous injuries. An hour and a half later, I was finished.

"Hey, Doc, thanks! My hand works as good as new!"

"You're welcome," I said.

"Can I leave now?"

"It's dark out now. I'm leaving the hospital, too. I'll walk you to your car."

■ Another non-ER story, but it's sufficiently bizarre to warrant inclusion in this book.

As part of my training in psychiatry during medical school, I and the other students visited the State Center for Forensic Psychiatry, where they detain people who are judged to be criminally insane. As part of the tour of this facility, the staff gave two case presentations. I've totally forgotten one of the cases, but the other story was vividly impressed in my memory, and I'll never forget it. How could I?

Before his case was presented, Jack was introduced to the medical students. As he walked toward the front of the classroom, I noticed that his pants were falling down, and half of his derrière was protruding. No underwear, and it didn't seem to bother him. One of my friends whispered, "I think they've found the missing link." That may have been a tad overstated, but it's a good bet that Jack will never be asked to appear on the cover of *GQ* magazine. Unfortunately, his looks were his strong point.

Years prior, Jack had been at home with his mother, with whom he lived. For lunch one day, he made a peanut butter and jelly sandwich. Just after he finished making the sandwich, a man came to the door, asking directions. As he spoke with the visitor, Jack's Mom walked into the kitchen and took a bite from the PB&J sandwich. This enraged Jack, and he began stabbing his mother in the neck with the knife he'd used to make the sandwich. As blood spewed from her neck, some of it soaked the sandwich, which was now resting on the counter. After his Mom dropped to the floor, dead, Jack picked up the blood-curdled sandwich and began eating it as he walked toward the door. He resumed giving directions to the now-horrified visitor as if nothing unusual had happened, but the visitor beat a pell-mell retreat to call the police.

Somehow, I bet that Jack's jury had little difficulty buying his insanity defense.

■ "Everybody, feel sorry for me!" the patient screamed over and over again. Bart had been driving his motorcycle well over the speed limit on the freeway. That probably wouldn't have been much of a problem, but he happened to be traveling in the wrong direction. I was not surprised to learn that he'd been drinking beforehand.

Eventually, Bart's luck ran out and he plowed into an oncoming car. The violent impact separated him from his Harley, catapulting him a few hundred feet down the freeway. He was lucky that he wasn't killed—or was he? The impact broke his neck, which paralyzed his arms and legs.

As I began thinking of the things he'd never do, I *was* feeling sorry for him. He'd never walk again. He'd never make love again. He'd never even scratch his own back. Nor would he ever get drunk and ride his motorcycle, terrorizing and endangering the lives of hundreds of innocent motorists.

"Everybody, feel sorry for me!"

■ I was absolutely dumbfounded. I had called the obstetrician down to see a patient in the ER who was nearing the end of her pregnancy. When I examined her, I could see the scalp of her baby through her cervix, which was dripping pus. She'd sustained what is termed a premature rupture of the membranes. From the history, it seemed clear that this had occurred a couple of weeks prior. In the interim, the tissues surrounding the baby had become infected. This was obvious.

After the obstetrician examined the patient, he came out and announced that he was going to discharge her on oral antibiotics. *Discharge* her? On *oral* antibiotics? Over my dead body!

I seriously considered whether the elderly obstetrician was manifesting signs of Alzheimer's disease. But I was here to protect the patient, not his feelings. I couldn't admit the patient to that hospital, since he was the obstetrician on-call, so I transferred her to a nearby facility. I then wrote a note to the head of the obstetrics and gynecology department. No one likes being a snitch, but this malpractice could not be overlooked.

■ Deciding that a fast-food restaurant was as good a place as any for a gunfight, some gang members began firing at members of a rival gang. Spraying the inside of the McDonald's® with hundreds of bullets from their Uzi® machine guns, they managed to kill their rivals, but they also injured several innocent bystanders as well. Typical Detroit marksmanship.

The victims were brought to the ER in which I was working. As I worked on one of the patients, I began speculating on how they would describe this event in the newspapers. Somehow, McDonald's® and guns seemed an incongruous mix. Then it hit me. "Call it the Big Mac Attack!" I exclaimed. This seemed to fit, and the name of this previously innominate battle spread around the ER. When the reporters arrived, they agreed it was a rather apt description, so that's how it became known. This name probably wasn't much of a hit at McDonald's® headquarters, though. I'm sorry, Ronald. I couldn't help myself.

■ Having worked in emergency rooms in both rich and poor areas, I am struck by one glaring dissimilarity: I've never seen a person in a poor area attempt suicide. I'm sure that some poor people try to kill themselves, but I just can't recall such a case. Put some money in someone's pocket, on the other hand, and they're swallowing handfuls of Tylenol®. Does this make sense? On the face of it, no.

Upon further reflection, I think this may simply reflect cultural differences in handling depression. In my estimation, I think that very few of the patients I saw who had attempted suicide actually wanted to die. I think most were just crying out for help, and some just lacked common sense—and may not have actually been trying to kill themselves. Melissa fit into the latter category.

"Hi, Melissa, how are you feeling?"

Trembling, she responded, "Uh-uh-uh, not good!"

"What did you take?" I asked.

"Caffeine pills."

"How many did you take?"

"Forty."

"*Forty?* Why so many?"

"Well, I was trying to study, and I felt tired and couldn't concentrate, so I took a couple of pills. They didn't do much for me, so I took some more."

"I see . . ."

". . . and some more. But it didn't help me much with my studying. And then I got jittery, and then I threw up."

"Melissa, didn't you read the directions on the bottle of caffeine pills?"

"Yes."

"And what did it say?"

"To take one or two pills, as needed."

"So why did you take so many?"

"Well, if two are good, forty are better, right?"

Obviously not. On another occasion, I had a virtually identical case in which a woman took a similar number of Tylenol® pills, reportedly because two pills just didn't give her the headache relief she sought.

■ The security guard sauntered back to the ER treatment area, telling one of the nurses that a visitor in the waiting room had collapsed, apparently having a seizure. Since most ER personnel possess a ho-hum attitude toward seizures, the nurse took her time getting there. When she finally arrived, she saw that the patient wasn't moving—or breathing, for that matter. This should have prompted the nurse to examine the patient more carefully and immediately institute therapy, but the nurse was still assuming that the guard's diagnosis of seizure was correct. Seizure = no big deal = I'll take my sweet time, thank you.

Eventually, the increasingly purple patient was brought to the treatment area. Seeing her as she was being brought in, I checked her ABCs (airway, breathing, circulation) and found that she had no pulse. I started the code, determining that she was in ventricular fibrillation (basically, her heart had stopped pumping), and defibrillated (shocked) her, thus restoring a normal rhythm. The patient lived. All's well that ends well, right? Usually, but I'm not quite that happy-go-lucky. I was aghast that the nurse would unquestioningly accept the guard's diagnosis, so I asked her to come into my office.

"Julie, you're a trained professional. You know much more than the guard, so you should have done your own assessment, and arrived at your own conclusions. It's dangerous to assume that a lay person has made the correct diagnosis."

She proclaimed, "But the guard said that she had twitched!"

Somewhat surprised that she didn't know the following tidbit, I explained, "It's not uncommon for someone to jerk at the onset of an arrhythmia (abnormal heart rhythm) which causes them to lose consciousness."

"Well, I thought it was a seizure!"

I asked, "Did you check for a pulse?"

"No, but . . ." Her eyes stared toward the floor. We both knew that she'd botched this one, and I'd made my point, so I let the matter drop. End of story? Not when fragile egos are involved.

Before I knew it, the head nurse was asking to speak with me. "What did you say to her?" she inquired.

I reiterated the original conversation. When the head nurse replied that Julie was in a back room crying her eyes out, I was shocked. "Why would she be so upset?"

"Well, Dr. Pezzi, she felt that you were hard on her."

"Hard on her? You must be joking. Julie is one of my best friends. I like her very much. I was about as hard on her as I would have been if I was explaining to my Grandmother that she had over-baked a batch of cookies. I simply explained that what she did was wrong. I certainly don't relish this part of my job, but I think it's my obligation to tell people when they make mistakes. That could have been my Mother or your Mother lying there in the waiting room, with her brain cells dying from a lack of oxygen."

"Well, I know, but she's upset . . ." And that she was, indeed. Julie seemed perpetually bitter after that day, and she soon transferred to another department. If you don't like the message, blame the messenger. If that doesn't work, just avoid the problem by avoiding the messenger.

Walking on eggshells is never easy, but it's especially difficult in an ER. Although I am embarrassed to admit this, I was pressured to eventually lower my standards so that I could harmonize with most of the nursing staff. Some of the nurses—especially the older, more experienced ones—were highly intelligent, competent, diligent professionals who performed flawlessly, but others were not about to accede to a perfectionistic doctor. They weren't shy about relaying this message to me, either. One nurse, who had been "laid off" from General Motors after repeatedly drinking on the job, challenged me to "step outside" for a fistfight. His emaciated frame didn't intimidate me much, but I didn't think it would look very good to have a slugfest in the ER parking lot. Besides, this twerp was drunk, and he was a *semi*-decent fellow when he wasn't plastered. Consequently, I declined his generous offer of an old-fashioned brawl. Nonetheless, I was rightfully worried about his on-the-job drinking, which was a regular thing for him. I relayed my concern to the nursing administrator who was in charge of the ER. This didn't go over well.

Ms. Pulchritude was a very attractive woman, at least until she opened her mouth. This administration's Golden Girl was despised by the nurses, hated by the doctors, and loathed by everyone else. Everyone, that is, except the hospital's CEO, who was rumored to be sleeping with her.

"So, you've said that you have smelled alcohol on his breath on several occasions. Do you have any proof that he was drinking on the job? I mean, did you see him do it?"

"No, but the smell is unmistakable." ER personnel don't even bother to guess whether or not someone has been drinking. We *know* if they have, and we bet on the patient's blood alcohol level (BAL). This is a regular form of entertainment in the emergency room, and the betting pools provide a nice supplementary income to those who are proficient in guessing the correct BAL.

I went on to explain that I thought he was drinking on his breaks and at lunch, since the smell of booze on his breath seemed much worse after those times. Clearly, this did not breech Ms. Golden Girl's sense of propriety, as she said, "*So?* What he does on his own time is *his* business, not *yours*!"

Wondering what planet she was from, I explained that alcohol does not miraculously disappear from the bloodstream after a 15-minute break. As I uttered this explanation, I wondered to myself why I was explaining this to someone who was, presumably, a nurse[25].

"What proof do you have? Do you know his BAL?"

---

[25]      Medical personnel might appreciate the following story, which further illustrates her almost unfathomable incompetence. On another occasion, Ms. Pulchritude called me into a conference room, and began berating me for ordering an ABG (arterial blood gas) on a patient complaining of shortness of breath who had been in a fire. Instead, the Leggy Wizard opined, I should have just done pulse oximetry (which measures the oxygen saturation of blood). I almost coughed up my lunch. This was tantamount to a first-year medical student telling the Chief of Surgery how to do an operation. Not only was I well aware of the limitations of a pulse oximeter (they can give incorrect readings in patients who've been exposed to carbon monoxide, and they don't measure the carbon monoxide content of blood), but I'd done research years ago, designing a device similar to a pulse oximeter which would measure the carboxyhemoglobin saturation (how much carbon monoxide is in the blood) in addition to providing a true reading of oxygen saturation. In short, this was right up my alley. Apparently not hers, though. Nonetheless, the lack of knowledge should never deter a dogmatic person from espousing their dogma. I explained that an ABG *could* measure the parameters that I wished to determine, unlike our pulse oximeter. "Well," she countered, "you didn't order an ABG on another patient who was in the same fire!" Duh, I thought. "Ms. Pulchritude, that other patient was exposed to the fire for a much shorter period of time, and he was without any symptoms or signs. It was a totally different situation." This not-very-minor point never sunk in, and she began yapping about how pulse oximetry would have been "good enough" for the first patient. "Good enough for what?" I wondered. To serve as incontrovertible proof of incompetence in a subsequent malpractice suit?

      As difficult as it may be to believe, this person was actually in charge of the ER and ICU at that institution, which was a large, teaching hospital. The Peter Principle? Or the Pulchritude Principle? Actually, considering her reputed relationship with the CEO, the first term is probably a bit more apropos—especially when taken as a double-entendre.

"No," I explained, "he wasn't exactly agreeable to having his blood drawn for an alcohol determination."

"You mean you *asked* him? He could sue you for libel!"

"Yes, I asked him, and he told me to go \*μ¢# myself. But it seems to me that he would be willing to prove he wasn't under the influence of drugs (which I also suspected, given his glassy-eyed stare and erratic behavior) or alcohol, if he had nothing to hide."

We were at loggerheads. She couldn't believe I was sticking my nose into his business, and I couldn't believe that she failed to understand that this was *not* a private matter. Who would want a drunk nurse working on them? The answer to this being obvious, I was stunned that she would abnegate her responsibility to investigate this matter. I wonder if hospital administrators can be sued for malpractice? No, of course not. They're immune to such a fray—and they know it.

■ Physicians who are not pathologists tend to view pathologists as being cast in a different mold, if not actually warped. Are they? You be the judge.

During medical school, I did a stint at a Medical Examiner's office in a major metropolitan area. I won't name it specifically, as I'm sure they wouldn't appreciate the publicity. The forensic pathologists at that facility had many tricks with which they entertained the impressionable young medical students under their tutelage. Foremost in my mind in this regard was the scrotal blowtorch demonstration.

After death, amazing amounts of flammable methane gas can accumulate in the body. In males, this sometimes considerably distends the scrotum. Had the pathologists simply explained that the captive gas was flammable, I would have believed them. Really. But no, they had to demonstrate. Spearing the scrotum with a huge needle, they'd ignite the escaping gas with a Bic® lighter (that's another Bic® commercial you will never see) and—voilà—instant blowtorch!

■ And now for another non-ER story that I whimsically decided to include . . . well, this *is* an ER story, but it pertains to animals. Animal lovers and the certifiably squeamish can skip this tale.

It's too bad that animal owners don't have to pass some sort of I.Q. test before they're allowed to own an animal. Had such a law been enacted years ago, this tragedy never would have occurred. As it was, it did. It was told to me by my girlfriend at the time, Stephanie, who was a veterinarian.

I can't recall what the original problem was, but the pet's redneck owner decided to bring his dog to the vet's office. He put the dog in the back of his pickup truck (what, you were expecting a Mercedes®?), and put a chain around the dog's collar. Unfortunately, the chain was far too long. Somewhere en route to the vet, the dog jumped out of the truck, and was dragged on the pavement. This erased a good deal of his skin, abrading down to—and through—muscle, tendons, and bone. The dog was admitted to the animal hospital, but was forcibly taken home the next day by Mrs. Redneck, who complained of how much such care would cost. I'm sure the poor dog died a miserable, lingering death. It probably would have been better to euthanize the dog, and his owners.

Had I been the doctor in charge of this case, things would have turned out differently. I tend to be an activist in cases like this (which did little to endear me to the administrators, no doubt), and I would have charged the Rednecks with animal cruelty. Quite the antithesis of the business maxim that "the customer is always right," but what the heck.

■ Another activist story. Telling you this story might get me killed some day because, as you will see, I helped to send four young men to prison for murder[26]. Had I not been working in the ER that night, they might have gotten off scot-free. But I'm getting ahead of myself. Let's step into the ER, and watch the story unfold.

"Dr. Pezzi, we need you in the radio room, stat." I'd heard parts of the paramedic's original transmission over the loudspeaker, and his mention that her heart had stopped sent me scurrying to the radio. The ambulance was on the scene of an automobile accident. A woman in her twenties was on her way to work in the evening, and she'd swerved to miss something. She lost control of her car, veered off the freeway, rolled over, and was ejected from the vehicle.

When she arrived in the ER, I noted that she had a large mark on her side, near the liver. On her way out of the car, she had struck the windshield pillar. I also noted that her abdomen was protruding, although she was slim. Clearly, she'd had a massive abdominal hemorrhage. When I checked her retinas with an ophthalmoscope, I was shocked to find virtually no blood in the retinal vessels. This didn't bode well for her survival, as it meant that her brain was similarly deprived of blood, and hence dead.

The combination of trauma and no heart beat is a virtual death sentence, but we give young people every possible chance to live. She did respond

---

[26]     In case they're seeking revenge after being paroled, I renewed my CCW license!

to the resuscitation, and I was able to obtain a good pulse and blood pressure. For the time, her body—if not her brain—was alive. The surgeon took her to the operating room, but the internal damage was too extensive. He tried valiantly, but she expired during surgery. I wasn't surprised. That she would die was a foregone conclusion; the only question was when it would happen. Knowing this, I'd already asked the next logical question.

*Why* had she swerved? Someone had thrown a Halloween dummy off an overpass. In the twilight, it might have appeared to be a person. Or, perhaps she didn't like the idea of smacking a dummy at 70 m.p.h., so she tried to avoid it. On to the next question.

*Who* had thrown the dummy off the overpass? The only witness to the accident, other than the perpetrators, was now dead, and there were no other clues. This senseless death angered me. For a time, it seemed as if the pranksters might get away with murder. I was determined to see that this did not happen.

When I was a resident training in Detroit, there was a case in which an ophthalmologist was killed by a bowling ball dropped off an overpass, and there were a number of other similar crimes in which there was no motive other than that which could be concocted by a malicious, sick mind. All of these cases remained unsolved. This one would be different.

I knew the key to solving this case was publicity. This couldn't be just another entry in the police blotter, it had to be Page 1 news. I began by calling the hospital's publicist. I asked her to contact newspapers, and television and radio stations to get the story out. When I got home in the morning, I did the same.

The media did a great job, publicizing this case to the hilt, which eventually resulted in the apprehension of the criminals. Earlier, I had speculated as to who might have done such a thing. I suspected that it was committed by a couple of 13 to 15-year-old boys, but I was wrong. They ranged in age from 19 to 22, which shocked me. Men (?) that age are usually obsessed with jobs, education, sports, polishing their car, drinking beer, and getting laid—*not* with puerile Halloween pranks.

■ And now a story from the "*What* were you *thinking?*" department. An 18-year-old guy was helping a friend work on his car, which had stalled on a freeway exit ramp at night. Tragedies are often rooted in a concatenation of errors, and this was no exception. While the friends tinkered with the car, a drunk driver zipped by in a pickup, pasting one of the friends on his grille. Without stopping, he drove exactly two miles, parked his truck on another freeway exit ramp, and walked home. When the truck stopped, the body peeled from the grille, and slumped to the pavement. This was noticed by a passerby, who called 911.

In the ER, we did emergency intrathoracic (inside the chest) surgery, to no avail. I'm sure the kid was dead as soon as he was hit, but ER doctors tend to be very aggressive in trying to revive young people. Had the drunk driver summoned help immediately, the outcome may have been different. Probably not, but one never knows. Hence the rationale for laws against hit-and-run accidents.

Surprisingly, cases in which an intoxicated driver leaves the scene of an accident are common. I suppose they're trying to avoid being caught while they are drunk, but they might just be in too big of a hurry rushing to the next bar to bother with anything so trivial as an injured human being. Who knows? Trying to understand what goes on inside the mind of a drunk is always problematic. Nevertheless, parking a blood-drenched car on a freeway exit ramp? What, he thought the police would never trace the car to him? *Duh!*

▪ A middle-aged couple were camping at a nearby campground. In the middle of the night, the woman got up for a drink, ostensibly to quench her thirst. Instead of water, she gulped down turpentine. Not exactly my choice of the ideal nightcap . . .

The husband's game plan was simple. Detox the little woman, and it's back to good ol' Jellystone Park for a yabba-dabba-doo time. Ever the spoilsport, I said no. It seemed a tad odd to me that a middle-aged woman would ingest a large amount of turpentine. You know, different smell, different jug, different taste—and she didn't even spit it out. This she attributed to being tired. I didn't buy it. I spoke with the on-call psychiatrist, and he was equally skeptical, so he admitted her. This brought forth howls of protest from the couple, who vehemently denied that she was suicidal. Perhaps, but my "incredulometer" was pegged, and it wouldn't let me believe her explanation. Besides, one good burp by the campfire and who knows?

▪ Another distilled beverage anecdote. A craggy-faced alcoholic was brought to the ER near death. The boozer had consumed far more whiskey than even he was accustomed to, and he was about two sips away from that great distillery in the sky. Ours was not to reason why, so we saved his life.

The paramedics who'd transported the man to the hospital had kindly chosen to bring along what remained of his supply of spirits. There, tucked neatly beside his leg, was a half-empty fifth of whiskey. I can't remember the brand, but it wasn't something I'd drink. A nurse dumped the liquor down the drain, and threw the bottle in the trash. Word of this deed eventually reached one of the administrators, who threw a conniption fit. The administrator said the whiskey was private property, and that the nurse had no right to discard it. He insisted that the alcoholic, upon his discharge from the hospital, be given a note of apology and a new fifth of whiskey.

Knock, knock, *hello*, Mr. Administrator, is anybody home? You want to give more booze to a man who almost drank himself to death? Hey, and the next time someone survives after shooting themselves, should we take them out to a gun shop and buy them another box of bullets, too?

▪ Nitrous oxide (a.k.a., laughing gas) is frequently used in the ER to provide relaxation and to relieve the pain of certain procedures. Occasionally, we give it to the patients, too.

A person whose brain is numbed by nitrous is apt to say and do things they wouldn't ordinarily say or do. In that regard, the effect of nitrous is similar to that of alcohol. Sometimes a person will giggle uncontrollably, which is why they call it laughing gas. Other nitrous-facilitated behaviors include a compulsion to say things that are better left unsaid. For example, one fellow issued a rather lengthy critique of a certain nurse's physique, describing to her all of the flaws that he was able to perceive. Consequently, he was automatically disqualified for our Favorite Patient of the Week Award.

Susan was equally outspoken. As I prepared to reduce her dislocated patella (i.e., push her kneecap back in place), she said, "I'm getting wet." I assumed that her IV was leaking, but I checked it, and it was fine.

I then guessed that she had spilled some urine, and I said that I'd send a nurse in to help her with that. "No, I'm getting wet *down there!*"

"Yes, I know," I responded, "I'll have a nurse step in."

"No, silly, it's not my *bladder*—it's my *vagina!*"

▪ Boris immigrated to the United States from Russia, or the USSR, or the former Soviet Union, or whatever they're calling it these days. He complained of having blood in his urine, so the nurse instructed him to go into the bathroom, void in a urinal, and then bring the urinal out with him. He looked surprised, telling the nurse that he found her request to be bizarre. The nurse assured him it was a routine request, and something which was essential to his evaluation. He walked into the bathroom with a puzzled look of cross-cultural disbelief.

A minute or so later, we heard some loud noises emanating from the bathroom. I thought he was having a seizure, so I opened the door to the bathroom. I yelled, "Boris, **what** are you doing?"

He replied, "The nurse told me to pee in the urinal, and then to bring the urinal out with me." Good ol' Boris had been trying to rip the urinal off the wall!

I said, "Not *that* urinal!" I pointed to the plastic urinals on the shelf, saying, "Use one of *those* urinals."

■ Carol was a hospital volunteer, what people call a "candy striper." And yes, you salivating maniacs out there, she was gorgeous. Beautiful, slim, intelligent, personable—but a high school student. She told me that she wanted to go to nursing school so that she could become a trauma nurse. Hearing this, I thought that she might want to see some trauma, and she eagerly accepted.

I knew it was best to start with something minor. I had a patient with a cut on his head which required suturing. I asked if she would like to watch me do the repair, and she agreed. I stationed her on the side of the stretcher that was opposite me.

As the procedure progressed, I explained everything as I went along. Since that was a teaching hospital and I was the teacher, this seemed perfectly natural. As I began explaining something, I looked at her and noticed that she was pale. Her eyes were half-closed, and she didn't respond when I said her name. Knowing what was about to happen, I raced over to her. Just as I got behind her, she passed out and fell backward, knocking me over. I didn't want to touch her with my bloody gloves, so I held my hands out laterally, still using my elbows to keep her from falling to either side. Her head came gently to rest on my chest, instead of smashing into the floor. I called for help, and a nurse came in to help her get up. I changed my gloves and finished suturing, alone.

While this may not have been an auspicious beginning, I've seen many doctors faint the first day of anatomy lab, so her career plans were not necessarily finished. So, Carol, did you become a trauma nurse? (I know that Carol isn't your *real* name, but . . .)

■ When I was about twenty feet away from the door to his room, I was struck by an overwhelming stench. This wasn't the usual fetid ER smell; this was worse. Far worse. Something was rotting in that room.

I entered the room and introduced myself. As the patient spoke, I realized that his mouth was the source of the odor. He reeked so intensely that I felt faint. Still, I had to do my job. I had to examine his mouth.

I'd never before—or since—seen anything like this. His teeth were rotting spindles, each coated with about a ¼-inch thick layer of plaque. Some of these stalactites would wobble when he would speak, and several had obviously already fallen out. His gums were red and raw, oozing pus, which pooled in his mouth. I felt his forehead; he felt hot, very hot. In the lingo of the ER, he was septic, and his mouth was the nidus of the infection. I admitted him for IV antibiotics, and to see a dentist, of course.

■ I have found that most people are curious as to whether or not physicians are attracted to members of the opposite sex. It's possible, but it doesn't happen as often as you might imagine, especially in an ER. Attractive women are as rare as dodo birds in emergency rooms. After a decade of ER work, I can recall having had less than a dozen attractive female patients. Considering the countless thousands of patients that I've served, this fact is truly amazing and deserving of formal study. A considerable amount of money is spent every year on the research and prevention of accidents, yet I've never seen anyone look into the reasons why attractive women seem to be virtually immune to diseases and accidents that might cause them to need emergency medical treatment. An intriguing phenomenon, to be sure, but perhaps I am skirting the issue (pun intended). Assuming that a single, attractive woman *did* show up in the ER, would I ask her out for a date? Not in this day and age. If she wanted to date me, she would have to be the one to do the asking *and* she would have to be content with a platonic friendship until I could trust her implicitly. In all of my years of training, no professor or sage even mentioned whether it's permissible to date someone that you met in the ER. Lacking the ability to learn by osmosis, and fearing the medical Gestapo, I feel more comfortable avoiding this matter altogether. Relying upon common sense, it seems to me that it is obviously taboo to date women whose medical care required an intimate exam, such as a pelvic exam. On the other hand, I see no reason why a woman with a finger cut should be subject to the same exclusion. ER doctors that work in small towns will, sooner or later, treat almost everyone in the area. If all women patients were perpetually off-limits, such ER doctors would either have to marry early, forgo marriage, or get a mail-order bride. Some choice.

■ Off to see my next patient. Walking into the room, I was struck by the incongruity of her presence. She was beautiful, and somehow she managed to penetrate the invisible force-field that seemingly keeps attractive women out of emergency rooms[27]. Her silky, slim, and tanned legs were enticingly framed by shorts that were, well, short. As I walked toward her left side, her lithesome trunk twisted in synchrony, tugging at her shirt, exposing a taut abdomen which had obviously never seen the bottom of a bag of Cheetos®. She tossed her head back, sending hundreds of curls dancing in a sensuous swirl. Her eyes gleamed with libidinous ardor, and she flashed a smile that was friendly, yet inviting. She wasted no time in announcing that she was single, which led me to conclude that she was half-blind, and had mistaken me for Tom Cruise. She came to the ER because she accidentally cut her hand with a knife, and when I moved in closer, I knew why. Her breath reeked so strongly of alcohol that my eyes began to sting . . .

The preceding two paragraphs were excerpted from my book, *Fascinating Health Secrets*. (Although the two excerpts from it which are presented in this book might suggest otherwise, that book is primarily a collection of health tips.) Interestingly, no one has applied for the $1000 prize. Perhaps my asseveration (about there being an inverse correlation between a woman's beauty and the likelihood that she'll be a patient in an ER) is not as flip or as baseless as it might seem.

▪ For a variety of reasons, we try to discourage patients from walking around the ER. However, some are too nosy—or bored—to comply with such a request. One lady meandered into the trauma room, and came out of the room as I was walking by its door. In a huff, she said, "Well I never! That man in there was *so* rude! I just tried making some conversation, but he wouldn't answer me. Wouldn't even look at me! How rude!"

I replied, "Ma'am, the man in there isn't *rude*. He's *dead*."

▪ I was performing a mental status examination on George, who had sustained a head injury. (This is a test to determine whether or not all of the lights are switched on upstairs.)

**Dr. Pezzi:** Who is the President?

---

[27]     ***Want to earn up to $1000?*** I'll put my money where my mouth is. If you're a beautiful woman, and you've actually been a patient in an emergency room, I'd like to hear your story. Burst my bubble of incredulousness and make money at the same time! Send your anecdote, and a picture of yourself, to the address listed at the end of this book. Now, for the fine print of the contest:

THE FINE PRINT. (1) The amount of the payment shall be related to: **a)** how interesting the story is, **b)** whether or not you authorize me to include a description of your tale in future editions of this book and other publications by this author, **c)** the degree of your pulchritude, *and* **d)** the literary quality of your narrative. (2) All decisions of the judge (that's *me*) are final, and the judge shall be the sole arbiter of all awards. That said, I'm surprisingly fair, and generous! Now, take your shot at $1000 . . .

**George:** Of what company?

**Dr. Pezzi:** No, who is the President of the United States?

**George:** (long pause) Washington.

**Dr. Pezzi:** No, who is the current President?

**George:** Lincoln.

**Dr. Pezzi:** What is the sum of 2 + 2?

**George:** 2.

**Dr. Pezzi:** What was your mother's maiden name?

**George:** She never had one.

**Dr. Pezzi:** She never did?

**George:** No, she was never a maid.

George's sister then interrupted us. "You'd better ask him some easier questions, Doctor. He wouldn't have known the answers to those questions even before he hit his head."

■ Mark and his family were visiting his boss at home on a Saturday evening. Brooke, Mark's 4-year-old daughter, was playing in the backyard when the boss' pit bull attacked her. After Mark kicked the dog repeatedly, the dog finally relented, and Brooke was taken to the ER.

I've seen many people mauled by dogs, and a disproportionate number were inflicted by pit bulls. This was especially true in the case of the severe maulings in which people were ground into hamburger—not just bitten once or twice. When I first saw Brooke, my heart sank. Her legs were shredded, with huge flaps of skin torn off in several places. A thousand stitches or so later, her legs would be a patchwork of scars. In spite of hours of plastic surgery, they would never be anything she'd want to show off at the beach, or even to her husband some day. Such a disfiguring injury would, I'm sure, cause her untold hours of anguish. I knew this, and so did Mark. He went home, got his gun, and went to the scene of the tragedy. There was the pit bull, still licking its lips, as if it had just eaten a tasty bowl of meat. Mark leveled his gun on the dog, and blew it into kingdom come.

■ It's clear that this lady needed help, but after seeing her, so did I. She was in her late thirties, dressed in an Army camouflage outfit, and reeked of cigarette smoke. Paraphrasing her story would not do it justice, so I'll present it verbatim.

"I knew I hated you the minute I saw you! I have the right to like who I want, and you're not one of them. I do not care to associate with you. Hey, I want to see someone from AA. If they have you committed, will they make you take your medicine? I'm disabled and on Medicaid. I want to have a smoke. I'm going outside. My Dad died of lung cancer, and they had to operate on him. I want to see Mental Health. Hey, stupid, are you Mental Health? M-e-n-t-a-l h-e-a-l-t-h, I spelled it for you, 'cause you're probably too frigging dumb to know what it is. And where is my cigarette? My lawyer says I can smoke whenever I want to. He says that the addiction is part of my disability, which is protected by the Disability Act. So where's my cigarette? I got a note from my doctor, and I presented it to President Clinton and the Congress. I'm going to be a nurse some day, or maybe a doctor—I haven't decided. I was supposed to take a test, but I didn't have the money for it. My smart-ass psychiatrist said that I'm mentally impaired. Now why would he say that? I told him to go f--- himself. He says I've got ADD. You know, hyperactive. What a bunch of crap. I'm on my way back from Wyoming. I drove out there in my motorhome. When I was there, they treated me like I was a piece of garbage. This doctor out there, he starts in on me like I'm some mental case or something. And I know what you're wondering—no, I haven't committed suicide. But you think I'm deranged, don't you?"

That was my first five minutes with her. Before I left the ER a few hours later, she'd punched me, hit me with a bottle, and tortured me with another hour of her harangue. Apparently I wasn't the only one whom she'd alienated. Spray painted on the side of her motorhome (incidentally, how could she afford it?) was the message, "Crazy woman get out of Wyoming. And don't come back. *Please*."

■ One glance told me that Ken had a fractured wrist. I asked him how it had happened.

"I was sitting on my roof . . ."

"You were *sitting on your roof*? Why?"

"I just like to go up there at night and be by myself," he responded.

"So how did you break your wrist?"

"Well, some kids walked by and started calling me 'dummy'."

"Yes, and then what?" I asked.

"I started to go after them, but I forgot I was on the roof, and I fell off."

# Role reversal

■ Like most people in my profession, I avoid doctors like the plague. I haven't had anyone I could call "my doctor" since I was a kid. Consequently, I don't have much experience as a patient. However, I did experience a shocking event with my Aunt when she was in an ER last summer. You would think I'd seen it all after working in emergency rooms for over a decade, but I hadn't.

My Aunt was dying of cancer. After experiencing massive internal bleeding, she was transferred to an ER (incidentally, not one in which I'd worked). After being there an hour or so, she became semi-coherent and anxiously agitated. Clutching her chest and thrashing about on her stretcher, she began screaming, "I can't breathe! I can't breathe! My chest hurts! I'm going to die!"

I went to the nursing station to inform them of this change in her condition, then I walked back to comfort her as best as I could. Since they weren't particularly busy, I expected that someone would soon be in to help. I was wrong. This puzzled me. They knew I was an ER doctor, and it would be reasonable to expect that they might give a shred of credence to my report of her condition, but no. They didn't come, so I went out to the nursing station once more. This time, a nurse did come, but he didn't seem particularly interested. I went back to holding my Aunt's hand, assuming he'd initiate basic interventions. Wrong again. Seeing that he was in no hurry to do anything, I suggested, "How about giving her some oxygen?"

He was in an argumentative mood. Dourly, he replied, "We checked her pulse ox (pulse oximetry, which measures the blood's oxygen saturation), and it's OK."

I explained to him that the pulse oximetry reading in my Aunt may have been factitiously high, and that breathing pure oxygen would increase her blood's oxygen content at least somewhat, and thus be of benefit to her. He seemed angered by this. Reaching for an oxygen mask, he threw it at me, striking my left arm. He commanded, "*You put it on her!*"

Quite taken aback by his overt hostility and insolence, I thought, "Hey, I'm here to comfort my Aunt, not to be a member of the ER staff!"

I then suggested doing an EKG. Another quarrel. "We already did one, uh, I think." With this, he began shuffling through her chart.

Wondering what the heck he was doing, I said, "Her condition has changed appreciably. Even if one was done earlier, there is now an indication for repeating it." He didn't like this suggestion, and told me that he would need an order for it. I thought this was odd, since I've never worked in an ER in which nurses could not perform an EKG at their own discretion. I also thought it was strange that he seemed so resistant to all of my suggestions. As a professional courtesy (and for their own self-interest, if nothing else), medical personnel typically accede to such requests from a family member who is a physician, especially when the suggested intervention is benign. What's the big deal about doing an EKG? It's not as if I were ordering their surgical team to prepare the operating room for stat open heart surgery, which I planned to perform myself.

Later on, I asked to see her lab results, but I was refused . . . surprised? Technically, they were within their rights to do that, but again it was a breach of etiquette. There's an unwritten rule that family member MD's can be made privy to test results. Whenever I was the ER physician in such a situation, divulging this information was unquestioningly the right thing to do. I think people possess an innate sense of propriety, and not to keep medical professionals in the family posted with the lab and x-ray findings is unnecessarily cruel. Besides, if they're kept informed, they might offer useful suggestions. No physician knows everything, and any physician who isn't willing to at least consider a suggestion is a fool.

Without going into too much detail, as time progressed I noticed that the staff were not attentive to various not-very-minor aspects of her care. Mentioning these, I was met with still more resistance. When I was working in the ER and a family member mentioned that something was wrong, I'd either thank them for the information or, at the very least, acknowledge it and say that I'd take care of it. But not these folks, who were one extremely unhappy crew.

Mentioning these events to a friend of mine, I said that I was considering writing a letter to the president of that hospital. He assured me this would not do any good. He had served on a board with the hospital president, and knew what he was like: an arrogant, abrasive jerk. Rather than reprimanding his employees for their conduct, he'd probably have given them a pat on the back. I never wrote the letter.

# *So you want to be an ER doctor?*

■ Those who have read this book might assume that I didn't like being an ER physician.  For the most part, that's true.  Dealing with vulgar, screaming drunks, junkies trying to dupe me into giving them narcotics, repeated death threats, constantly changing sleep schedules, not having the time to eat or use the restroom, not seeing family and friends on holidays, smelling patients who hadn't bathed in months, moronic administrators, patients abusing the ER by coming to it for obvious non-emergencies (a mosquito bite, farting, a bad hair perm, a pimple, a questionably loose vagina, etc.), patients *screaming* "I'll sue you" to an innocent registration clerk within ten seconds after entering the ER—it all takes its toll.

Ever try to run three codes (cardiopulmonary resuscitations) at once?  I have, and you don't know what pressure is until you have.  It's commonly accepted that a human cannot be in more than one place at a time, but ER physicians are expected to be immune to this limitation.  If all patients who are being coded—*and **every** other patient in the ER*—are not treated as if they were the only person in the ER at that time, the doctor faces the very real possibility of a lawsuit.  Realistically, ER physicians can be flooded with more patients at one time than they can optimally care for, but this fact is legally irrelevant, and cannot be used in their defense.

Imagine that you're a cashier in a supermarket, and a dozen customers with overflowing grocery carts come into your line, in addition to the ones who were already there.  Imagine that you could be *personally* sued (losing your home, your car, money for your children's education and Christmas presents, and future wages) if you didn't check everyone out as fast and as flawlessly as you usually do.  No, you can't simply make them stand in line and wait their turn.  The analogy to ER is that some patients cannot wait; a patient who isn't breathing can't be scheduled for an appointment next Tuesday.

Imagine that one of the customers in your line, Mrs. Jones, has two carts full of groceries, a handful of coupons, and she must be checked out within the next four minutes—or else she can sue you, and she'll win.  You'd love to accommodate her, but Mr. Smith and Mrs. Clinton are demanding the same thing, too.  How would you feel if you were in this predicament?  If you think it is so impossible that no one would ever be expected to deal with it, you're wrong.  This is *exactly* the predicament which ER doctors find themselves enmeshed in every time the ER is swamped with critically ill patients—and that is not an uncommon event in an ER. If cashiers were subject to such potential liability, anyone who became a cashier must have rocks in their head. I feel the same about people who go into ER medicine.

The popularity of the television show *ER* might give *some* idea of the responsibility shouldered by an ER physician, but I doubt that it can adequately convey the pressure an ER doctor faces while working in a busy emergency room. For example, it is not at all uncommon for several patients to arrive almost simultaneously in the ER, virtually on their deathbeds. Each of these people might require extensive interventions—like CPR (cardiopulmonary resuscitation or "coding" someone), cardiac pacing, central venous line placement, and lumbar puncture—in addition to requiring intensive medical therapy. As the physician runs from patient to patient, he is often besieged by requests from nurses, ER assistants, residents, medical students, radiology technicians, patients, relatives of patients, paramedics, police officers, respiratory technicians, other physicians, hospital supervisors, and local TV stations and newspapers. Let's step into the ER for a few minutes . . .

> Nurse A shoves an EKG in my face, saying, "It's from the new guy they just brought in room 8; he's short of breath." The nurse scurries away, and I find that there is no chart for this patient. (Since that hospital had a policy against nurses taking verbal orders, it was incumbent upon me to assemble a chart so that I could begin writing orders on the patient. Great, I get to be a ward clerk, too.) Nurse B says, "The lady in room 12 is seizing, and we can't get an IV in her; the IV team tried, and they said that you'd have to do it." Nurse C demands, "When are we going to do the pelvic exam in room 10? The patient says she's tired of waiting." Nurse D informed me that the intoxicated, suicidal female patient in the Isolation Room walked out of the hospital three minutes ago. I requested the assistance of the hospital guard, and this insolent character had the temerity to refuse, saying, "Why don't *you* go get her?"[28] Nurse E tells me that the family of the patient in room 7 is

---

[28] One of the primary functions of hospital security personnel is to do the dirty work in restraining patients who are out of control, so that doctors can do just the doctoring, and nurses can do just the nursing. However, I had the misfortune of having a guard with a serious attitude problem (who, subsequently, had a serious employment problem). Since the doctor has the ultimate responsibility for all patients, regardless of who screws up, I went after the patient who, I found, had vanished into the winter night, and was never seen or heard from again. Administrators would like to believe that such problems either don't exist, or that they can just be turfed to the police. By the time the police arrive, though, it's often too late. In the case of the vanishing patient, we called the police within seconds, and they arrived within a few minutes, but by then the patient was long gone. Hence, the need for the doctor, the nurse, and the janitor to attempt interdiction when security guards are absent (or derelict). When I entered

*demanding* to see me **now**. The clerk announces, "Dr. M. wants to speak with you on line 1, and Dr. V. is on line 3; he's mad because he's been on hold."

Another person announces on the PA system, "Dr. Pezzi to the radio room stat!" (to give orders on a critical patient coming in by ambulance). The respiratory technician tells me, "I couldn't draw his ABG (arterial blood gas). Do you want to try?" The radiology technician wants me to look at a cervical (neck) x-ray of a trauma patient who is clamoring to get out of his neck brace and off the backboard. The Internal Medicine resident approaches me, asking me to discharge a patient from the ER that was seen by the prior ER doctor and referred to the Internal Medicine service for admission. That's a tough position to be in, as the chart dictated by the first ER doctor will undoubtedly stress the need for the admission (to palliate the Utilization Review Committee). If I discharge the patient, and the patient has an adverse outcome, I am a sitting duck for a malpractice attorney.

An ER staff member tells me that I should go examine the police prisoner in room 2 so that the guy can be discharged back to the prison; the patient realizes that it is more pleasant to be in a hospital than in jail, so he decides that he's having chest pain and screams, "And I'll sue you if you don't admit me!" The patient in room 4 leers at me whenever I walk by, eventually yelling out, "Hey, doc, I've been havin' this belly pain for three years. I want you to see me next!" The hospital public relations person is waiting to talk to me about three patients brought in with carbon monoxide poisoning; he tells me that Channel 12 wants to interview me ". . . when I get a minute." A psychiatric patient follows me around like a little puppy, saying, "I'm depressed. I'm suicidal. Admit me." I discussed this with the on-call psychiatrist, and he refused to admit the patient. He declared, "That person is just a junkie!" The mother of the patient in room 6 screams at me, "My child is *vomiting*!!!"

Imagine 15 minutes of this, with 10 hours to go until the shift is over. In reality, the scenario that I just depicted was even worse than how it was presented. For purposes of clarity, I relayed the dialogue from the first four nurses as if it occurred sequentially. Actually, those four nurses

the field of medicine, I never anticipated that I would one day be forced to function as a "step-in" security guard, and this is something I find abhorrent. The American legal system has given physicians who repudiate such a function a new title: that of "defendant." Given the choice between being a security guard and a defendant, I'll be a security guard. It's not a tough choice.

approached me at the same time and all four spoke simultaneously. After that, they darted away in unison, apparently complacent in their perfunctory discharge of their duty[29]. I immediately implored, "*Wait!* I cannot understand what you're saying when four people are speaking at the same time. You'll have to repeat your messages *one at a time.*"

Superficially, ER work may seem appealing: there's excitement, a steady paycheck, no need to invest in the practice, and no need to become involved in the business aspects of medicine (other than filling out an occasional insurance form).

On the other hand, the drawbacks of ER medicine are almost endless. In addition to the aforementioned factors, ER docs face:

- Frivolous lawsuits. Besides the suits generated when the ER is simply too busy for everyone to receive optimal care, ER physicians are often sued for no reason. Notice that I didn't say no *apparent* reason—I literally mean *no* reason. I have been sued when patients had perfect treatment and a perfect outcome. The fact that I was eventually dismissed from these cases didn't even the score. Each case cost me at least $5000 (for the *non*refundable malpractice insurance deductible) and untold hours of grief. How would you like it if someone could steal $5000 from you, and you would have no recourse? If this happened to more people in this country, I guarantee there would be a revolution. Do you think the UAW

---

[29]    Nurses inform the physician of critical patients and miscellaneous other hot potatoes because the physician, of course, must be apprised of such things. However, there is another pragmatic reason for such messages, and that's to pass the buck. After relaying the message to the doctor, they will dutifully write in the charts, "Dr. Pezzi informed." From a legal standpoint, any subsequent delay in attending to the now-documented problem makes it appear as if the physician were ignoring the issue. Yeah, right—I was sitting in my office, gawking at the *Sports Illustrated* swimsuit issue, callously ignoring the pleas from the nurses to help the patients.

When a nurse informed me of such a patient in a reasonable manner, I had no qualms with a subsequent notation that I was informed of the problem. That's just the nurse doing her job, and doing essential nurse CYA (they have to play that game, too). It's part of my job to shoulder the ultimate responsibility for the patients, and I am not objecting to this transfer of responsibility. What I *am* objecting to is when I'm "informed" in such a way (such as when four nurses spoke at the same time) that I was not truly informed at all. Not being dumbbells, the nurses must have realized that I could not comprehend four simultaneous messages. Nevertheless, they began walking away, apparently feeling that they'd discharged their duty. I've seen even worse behavior, though. Some nurses just chart that the doctor was informed without making *any* effort to inform the doctor. They don't care about the doctor or the patient, just themselves. But if there was a lawsuit in such a case, guess who would be sued? The nurse? *Of course not!* The dedicated nurse did her job and informed the doctor—or so she wrote in the chart. Yes, it's the ultimate scapegoat again: the *doctor* is the one who would be sued.

(United Auto Workers) would tolerate such an injustice to their members? It's inconceivable. The pusillanimous AMA (American Medical Association), on the other hand, doesn't even utter a peep.

• Countless subpoenas to appear as a witness. Bouncer **A** ejects unruly Drunk **B** from Bar **C**. Drunk **B** sues **A** and **C** for a sprained wrist or some other grave malady. The county prosecutor subpoenas the hapless ER doctor to appear as a witness. Typically, this occurs a few years after the incident, when the doctor has totally forgotten the patient. Realistically, all he can do is to serve as an unpaid reader of the chart, or serve as an unpaid expert. Failure to comply with the subpoena would result in the doctor being charged with contempt of court. Typically, these subpoenas are served on short notice, and they demand that the doctor appear in court at, say, 1 p.m. If the doctor worked the preceding night shift, that would fall right in the middle of his sleep time. How would you like to be forced to appear in court at 3 a.m.? I've had this occur as many as six times within a month (with the date of one trial being changed *four* times); if that wouldn't disrupt your schedule, what would?

• Being caught in *darned if you do, and darned if you don't* quandaries. It is generally accepted that complete documentation is a good thing for any doctor, and ER doctors in particular[30]. If we're sued, it's our best defense. At one hospital, I was recognized for having the best documentation of any ER physician. After moving

---

[30] Having seen some outpatient records, I am stunned by what passes as documentation for family doctors. For example, the chart for one visit simply said, "Sore throat." That's it. Was that the history or the diagnosis? Where's the examination? Was this a mild viral illness, or a person with an inflamed epiglottis—who could die within a matter of hours? Or was it referred chest pain—maybe the person was having a heart attack? Or maybe it was thyroiditis, and didn't involve the throat per se. What treatment was prescribed? In contrast, a typical ER chart for such a complaint could run over a page in length, typed with single spacing.

Family doctors can often get away with such shoddy documentation because their patients usually like them, and thus rarely sue. I've often been amazed by the incomplete examinations done by these doctors. For example, one young lady came to the ER complaining of abdominal pain. She had seen her doctor earlier in the day, and he couldn't determine the cause of her problem, so he prescribed Tylenol® and sent her home. The Tylenol® didn't help, so she came to the ER later in the day. After treating the patient, I called the physician to let him know what I'd discovered.

**Family doctor (FD):** Well, what did you find, Kev?

**Pezzi:** A 7½-pound baby boy. She was pregnant.

**FD:** She was *pregnant?!?*

**Pezzi:** Yup.

**FD:** Wow . . .

to another hospital, I wasn't praised for this, I was repeatedly criticized by the director of medical records. In attempting to slash her budget for transcription, she tried to coerce physicians into abbreviating their dictations. Anyone with any knowledge of medicolegal issues would know that this harebrained means of economizing was ludicrously shortsighted. Nevertheless, she was not to be dissuaded by such a fact, and—like an enraged pit bull—she kept on attacking. To his credit, my boss told her to buzz off, but she never stopped. Month after month, she would prepare charts, graphs, and statistical analyses of the cost of my dictations. She would fire off ranting memos to the hospital vice-president, and this pea-brained pencil-pusher would write his own memos, laden with invective. Is this your image of being a respected doctor? Frankly, mass-murderers are often hassled far less, and treated with more dignity.

Another example of this phenomenon occurs when doctors are hassled to do fewer labs and x-rays in order to save money. While I generally agree with cost-containment measures, one cannot overlook the fact that such tests are often the only means that a physician has of covering his butt and avoiding million-dollar judgements against himself. Realistically, society cannot coerce doctors into doing fewer tests, and then penalize them in a subsequent malpractice suit for not doing those tests. Realistic or not, this is just what is currently happening to American physicians. One of my former colleagues succumbed to this pressure, and decided against doing a CAT scan on a middle-aged man complaining of back pain. As it turned out, the man had an aortic aneurysm and died a day later. Had the CAT scan been done, he might have lived. Another former colleague saw a 30-something-year-old woman complaining of chest pain. Given her histrionic presentation, the patient's complaints seemed more rooted in neuroses than in reality, so she didn't do any tests. The patient died of a heart attack a day or two later. Any Monday-morning quarterback could see that these were two cases in which tests should have been done, but hindsight is always perfect, isn't it? It requires absolutely no skill, either, but it does allow for some pompous and self-righteous grandstanding. The only way to circumvent these occasional tragedies would be to thoroughly test everyone, but this is something we cannot afford. Life isn't perfect, and the imperfections of life sometimes put life at peril.

Given the amount of chaff that they're presented with, ER doctors do an amazingly good job of separating the wheat from the chaff. I couldn't even begin to tell you how many patients I've had who claimed to be paralyzed, yet were totally fine. Some of them had fooled me so convincingly that I had to drag a neurologist into the ER in the middle of the night. In each of these cases, the neurologist would put the patient through an exhaustive examination, and find nothing wrong. As the patient dressed and walked out of the ER, the neurologist would begin muttering how "that *µ¢#!$& patient cost me 3 hours of sleep!"

Some people wonder why doctors don't just run tests on the patients who *need* to have tests performed. Alas, this would require a crystal ball. Some patients are incredibly stoic, and adamantly deny that there is anything wrong. Should we subject these patients to a polygraph (lie detector) examination? Conversely, other patients profess to be dying, even when they are totally healthy. I've had days in which every ER patient was chaff, from an ER standpoint.[31] Imagine sorting through thousands of such cases per year, and being expected to never err. Quite literally, it's an unrealistic expectation.

• Dealing with "Quality Assurance" committees (QACs). To begin with, QACs—like most other government-mandated misnomers—have very little to do with quality. Their primary function is to harass doctors with inane trivialities. For example, most of the QAC issues I faced resulted when I was forced to explain why I didn't do this or that. So, I'd pore over the patient's chart and—*surprise!*—find that I *did* indeed do the thing in question. Then I'd have to draft an official response to the committee (which, in reality, is often just one person who can't find more gainful employment). After this happened a dozen or so times, I began recommending remedial reading lessons for the QAC reviewer. This did little to enhance my popularity with the "committee" and, thus piqued, they'd attack all the more, like any good bureaucrat. The expected response was to meekly and repentantly acquiesce, flagellating oneself for such an egregious error, and thanking the committee for its grand insight and wisdom.

---

[31]    I'll give an example. One fellow came to the ER by ambulance, complaining of chest pain. To make a long story short, he finally admitted that he wasn't having any problems at all, except that his car wouldn't run. He wanted to visit his girlfriend in the hospital, and he didn't have the money for a cab, so he called 911 for an ambulance ride. After we discharged him from the ER, the smiling love-struck man went to see his girlfriend, oblivious to his waste of $1500. (Of course, he had no insurance, so the taxpayers were stuck with that bill.) Such an execrable insouciance!

In short, they wanted you to take it up the rear, and then thank them for the attention. Kowtowing to incompetents is just not something I'm able to do. So the fight went on. What a waste of time and money.

I could go on and on, and fill an entire book with such drawbacks. Suffice it to say that anyone who decides to go into ER medicine, having been apprised of these factors, is certifiably insane or a masochist. In summary, if you want to go through life like a dog with his tail stuck between his legs, be an ER doctor. If there is another career in which a person is made to be more of a scapegoat for the collective shortcomings of society and simple reality, I'll eat my words—literally. This book, on national TV, anywhere.

In reality, I think many physicians *are* true masochists. This stems from their years in medical school and residency in which they were abused, and any protestation on their part was strictly forbidden. In fact, the expected response was not to remain silent, but to thank the person dishing out the abuse. For example:

**Psychopathic Professor of Surgery (PPOS):** Dr. Miller, what's the latest potassium on the patient in bed 462-B?

**Dr. Miller:** Uh, I'm sorry, I don't know. I sent the specimen to the lab two hours ago, but I just got out of surgery with Dr. Burns . . .

**PPOS:** *What?!?* You don't know the potassium?

**Dr. Miller:** (meekly, eyes gazing toward the floor) Uh, no . . .

**PPOS:** Well, if you don't know, *then who the h@## knows?*

**Dr. Miller:** Uh . . .

**PPOS:** Look you little S.O.B., you are *not* to waste my time on rounds like this in the future. You are to know *everything* about *every* patient, and I don't want any more lame excuses! Do you hear me?

**Dr. Miller:** Yes, Doctor. I promise that this won't happen again. I apologize for the trouble I've caused you. Thank you for bringing this matter to my attention.

And this is the PPOS on her good days. On her bad days, she actually physically assaulted residents. Sure, the residents could have turned her in for such abuse, but her fellow Psychopathic Professors would have just retaliated against the whistleblowers in other ways. So, the residents learned to keep mum, no matter what. They're well-trained. Care to join the club?

■ The tension was thick, but I didn't know why. This family hated me. They were seething, and they had just arrived. The patient was in his mid-twenties and claimed to be disabled. He still lived at home with his parents, who were also disabled, or so they said. These "disabilities" were shams, the type of which are lambasted in the press as being a flagrant waste of taxpayer's money. These people could have worked, but they chose not to. Three disability checks every month can buy one heck of a nice trailer home and pickup truck, so why work?

I tried to be courteous, but I was having as much luck wending my way out of this one as would a black man at a KKK rally. I realized the aptness of this analogy: it didn't matter who I was, or what I was like as a person. I had been dehumanized, and they couldn't see beyond the object of their prejudice. In this case, it wasn't the skin, it was the white coat. My doctor's smock. They hated me because I was a doctor.

The first tangible evidence of this hatred surfaced when "pa" muttered, "You &*!!@#~ doctors make too much money!" I think that our income is commensurate with the education and sacrifices necessary to become a physician, and I did not feel obliged to justify my salary. I've met people who make as much money mowing lawns in the summertime as I did working all year as a physician, but something told me that he would not harbor such resentment toward them. It's the old nonsensical class warfare thing: you got your money by stealing from the poor folks. You have more than us, so you must have cheated someone to get it. Haven't they ever heard of hard work? At that point in my life, even though I was only around 35, I'd already worked about as many hours as would an average man in a lifetime. I'd worked hard, and I wasn't about to suck up to an ungrateful maggot. Rather than outwardly bristle with indignation, I simply went on with my job. This peeved him all the more.

The security guard then asked "pa" to move his truck, which he'd parked in the spot reserved for emergency physicians. Having a reserved parking spot was one of the few perks of being an ER doctor; in fact, it's the only perk I can recall. The ER doc coming on for the next shift had requested that the vehicle be moved so that he could park his car in his assigned spot. That was too much for "pa" to swallow. The bleeping doctor wants to park in his assigned spot? Why, such gall! Nope, "pa" couldn't sit down for this one. Them was fightin' words, and "pa" was in the mood for a fight! He walked to his truck and opened the *passenger's* side door, smashing it into the side of my car, denting it. Such nonsense. This was witnessed by the security guard, who said that it was obviously intentional.

Now I was mad. I called the police and filed a police report, which I felt eminently justified in doing. The county prosecutor was outraged, and agreed to prosecute "pa." The administration of the hospital was equally outraged, but not at "pa." They were mad at *me* because I had the temerity to prosecute good ol' "pa." They didn't think this would make for good PR for the hospital. Tough luck, I said, I'm going to prosecute anyway. I gave them the chance to pay for the dent repair, but they refused. Fine, I'll just assert my right as an aggrieved person and prosecute him. The hospital brass felt that the behavior of patients and patient's families should be condoned, no matter what. Would police departments condone the malicious destruction of their officer's private property? No. Would a lawyer let you smash his car and walk off scot-free? Or would a high school student, for that matter? No. So what is it about people who deliver medical care that requires them to be defenseless targets? If there's a logical nexus here, I just don't get it.

■ Reminiscing about my years in the ER, I sometimes muse about the victories—the things I did which really made a difference. I'd guess most people would assume that CPR (cardiopulmonary resuscitation, or "coding" someone) would be the most dramatic and satisfying event for an ER doc. At least for me, that's rarely true. To begin with, most patients who are coded end up dead. Those who live often have permanent brain damage, even when their code is expertly performed. Rejoice about this? Nah.

I've had some satisfying outcomes, though. A 45-year-old man with a history of kidney failure presented to the ER about long enough to tell us his name and a few details of his medical history, then his heart stopped pumping. I was speaking with him as he passed out. We began the code. Not having any lab tests to rely on, I guessed that his blood's potassium level was too high, which can indeed cause the heart to stop. Unfortunately for doctors—and fortunately for lawyers—the practice of medicine is not as simple or as clear-cut as it may seem with the benefit of hindsight. This case was complicated in that he had kidney failure, which made him prone to a high potassium level, but he also possessed other factors which might cause his potassium to be decreased. Of the two, I thought it was more likely that his potassium was high, so I immediately began treating him for this. As I waited for the lab to determine his potassium level, I was concerned about the legal repercussions of a wrong guess. While no physician—except for those whose opinions are warped by being paid $400 per hour as an "expert witness"—would ever say that I was wrong, an attorney would have no problem finding some physician who lacked enough compunction and knowledge to testify that I'd committed malpractice. All too often in American courts, "clinical judgement" is synonymous with "a legal crapshoot." Had I been wrong, I would have made some lawyer a very happy person. And a rich one, too.

Working in an ER, it's sometimes necessary to make a snap decision before all the facts are known. If you're right, you can pat yourself on the back. If you're wrong, the sharks will smell blood and attack. In this case, if his potassium was low or normal to begin with (this patient also had intrinsic heart disease, which could cause his heart to stop even if the potassium level was fine), an attorney would lambaste me for lowering his potassium. "Dr. Pezzi," he'd pompously say, "isn't it true that a low potassium level can cause someone's heart to stop? Or, if it's already stopped, wouldn't it make it more difficult to restart?" Attorneys craft their questions to paint a certain picture, not to arrive at the truth. Anyone who thinks otherwise is incredibly naive, or in elementary school. To answer these questions truthfully, I'd have to say "yes." I'd try to explain myself, but I'd be cut off. "A simple yes-or-no answer will suffice, Doctor." A simple answer will suffice only for a simpleton, but that's never dissuaded any attorney. "So," he'd continue, "his potassium level was not high, and you lowered it, thus contributing to his death." With this, he would dramatically stride toward the jury, imploring them to find me guilty. "Ladies and gentlemen of the jury . . . Dr. Pezzi has admitted that a low potassium level can contribute to death. And what did this Doctor do? He lowered the patient's potassium level."

Darn right I did. And you know what? 90 minutes later the patient was awake and talking with his wife. His potassium had been very high, as I suspected.

What about the spineless approach? That is, why didn't I wait until the lab results were back before making a potentially serious guess? Uh, do you mean why didn't I just shoot the patient? Lesson #1 for prospective ER doctors is "don't rely upon the unreliable." Determining a potassium should take minutes, not hours. But having learned that laboratories are unusually susceptible to Murphy's law, I decided not to wait. Good thing I didn't. In this case, the potassium wasn't known for a couple of hours. People who are coded for such a period of time share one remarkable similarity: they're all dead. Hoping to prevent such an outcome, I exercised my clinical judgement, cognizant of the fact that some gutless shyster might disparage my judgement as being rash.

Monday-morning-quarterbacks are never wrong, but they're always worthless.

- One of the true tests of whether or not an ER doctor is dedicated is whether or not he is willing to disimpact a patient. If you're squeamish, you'd better skip this.

Simply put, disimpacting a patient involves manually digging the feces from a person's rectum with a gloved finger or two. People who are elderly and/or paralyzed are particularly prone to fecal impactions, which can cause a great deal of agony (the bowel goes into spasm trying to expel the waste matter). The I'm-here-for-the-paycheck, not-the-patient type of doctors do one of two things: dump the procedure onto a nurse, or order the nurse to do an enema. With a true fecal impaction, enemas often don't work, and when they do, they take far too long to act. What patient wants to writhe in pain for an hour or two?

Anyone who isn't a coprophiliac would be disgusted by such a procedure, and I share their disgust. It's gross and far smellier than you might imagine, but someone has to do it. Years ago, I realized that very few nurses would perform a disimpaction, so I stopped asking them. I just do it myself. A more grateful patient is hard to find, and that's enough reward for me.

# *Happy Days in the ER*

I don't want to leave you with the impression that I've never had any enjoyable experiences in the ER. Far from it. In fact, I've had countless positive experiences that I'll treasure forever. While it's true that the negative events predominated, I'm not surprised by this skewing. Anyone whose mind isn't warped by LSD or some other hallucinogen can readily appreciate that an emergency room is not exactly a hotbed of joy. Nevertheless, the indomitable human spirit persisted. Amidst the shadows of gloom, cheery rays of light shined through. Here are a few of my favorites.

■ My greatest fear as an ER physician was losing a young patient. Losing any patient is always sad, but if an elderly patient died, I was consoled by the fact that they at least had the chance to live a full life. The death of a young person, on the other hand, is always an unmitigated tragedy.

When Jacqueline arrived in the ER, I was filled with dread. An asthmatic in her early twenties, she presented on an ambulance stretcher, comatose and purple-grey in color. My first thought was that she was going to die, if she hadn't already. She had previously been intubated (having a tube inserted in her windpipe) and was being artificially ventilated. She also had received multiple intravenous (IV) and inhaled treatments by the paramedic on her way to the hospital. In spite of all that, she was still not responding. I allowed myself five seconds to panic, then I got busy.

An hour later, she remained comatose, although serial ABG's (arterial blood gases, which measure how well the lungs are working) revealed a marked improvement in her respiratory status. Now stabilized, we transferred her to the ICU. In the hubbub of the ER, my attention turned to other patients.

A week or two later, a thank-you note appeared in my mailbox at the hospital. Jacqueline said that she was already at home, and feeling fine. I was joyous. I thank God that she was given the opportunity to live the remaining 60 or so years of her life. And, for whatever time I have left on this Earth, I will always remember her.

■ Simply transcribing this note (from a 12-year-old) would not have done it justice. So, here's a copy of it (her signature is obscured by digital pointellization [pixelation]):

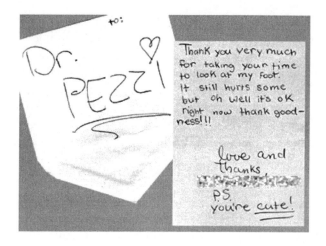

■ Another youngster was in the ER with one of her friends, and they sent me a couple of notes. One note read:

*Dear Kevin,*
*Thanks for helping me to get better.*
*Love,*
*Jessica*

Jessica's friend sent a note, too (I've interjected my comments in parentheses):

*Dear Pezzi,* (*Dear Pezzi?*—I love it!)
*Thanks for the wheelchair!* (I'd given them a wheelchair, more for amusement than anything else.) *Me and Jessica really appreciate it. And we apologize if we were a nuisance!!* (Nah, just playful! Actually, I was amused by their antics, but one of the nurses was not.)
*Love,*
*Mary & Jessica*

■ Soon after beginning a shift, I was told I had a phone call from a patient that I'd recently seen. "Dr. Pezzi, when you get home, I have a little present waiting for you on your porch." The caller, Mr. C., was one of the nicest people I've ever met in my life. An immigrant to this country, he was living proof that the route to success is hard work and determination, not a welfare check or a government subsidy.

At that time Mr. C. and I lived in the same neighborhood, and he knew the location of my home. When I arrived home in the morning, several large boxes were waiting for me. Opening them, I found a glass-topped patio table with a parasol, four padded patio chairs, an outdoor thermometer, and an outdoor ashtray. To put it mildly, I was stunned. What a pleasant—*and totally unexpected*—surprise! I was ebullient, but I wondered what it was I'd done to deserve such kindness. At the hospital the next day I asked Betty, who was a real sage and someone I respected immensely. "Well, Dr. Pezzi, it's obvious that he thinks very highly of you."

Years have passed since then, and every time I see the furniture I think of what Betty said, and I think of Mr. C.'s benevolence. It was truly touching. Kindness begets kindness, and I'm sure that at least a little bit of Mr. C.'s kindness rubbed off on me. With the cynicism engendered by a decade of ER work, it's true that no one will ever confuse me with Mother Theresa, but I'm trying.

■ Although I truly appreciated receiving such an expensive and useful gift as the patio furniture mentioned above, I've been given simple presents which were equally touching. Homemade jelly, bread, cake, pie, candy, and other delicacies were veritable treasures. I still exchange Christmas cards with some former patients, and that warms my heart, too. Others have sent me e-mail, thanking me and giving an update on their progress. Some have sent letters, all of which I still have and cherish. One young lady gave me a Pez® candy dispenser and some Pez® candy; considering my name, it was a great gift!

■ Another great reward was simply having the opportunity to interact with people. With the exception of those whose morals are impossibly at odds with my own, I like almost everyone. Rich or poor, educated or not, black or white, a corporate president or a garbage man (not that this is pertinent, but I've even given my garbage man a present . . . hey, they're people, too!)—no matter who you are, there is a good chance I'll like you. I've met professional athletes, movie stars, politicians, and other celebrities, but some of my most rewarding experiences came from having the opportunity to serve America's veterans. I think that too many people, their minds numbed by MTV and Baywatch, are oblivious to the debt we owe those veterans. The selfless sacrifices of the veterans are awe-inspiring, and I don't believe that our debt to them can ever be fully repaid. I was honored to be able to serve them. This summer, after mowing my lawn, I'm going to mow the lawn of a veteran who can't walk. If you're wondering whether or not I have anything better to do with my time, I can tell you forthrightly: the answer is "no."

▪ Life's simple pleasures are the best. Ordinarily, I wouldn't count the beginning of a shift in the ER as one of my favorite memories, but I've had some wonderful experiences at those times. Occasionally, a nurse would grab me and give me a big, warm hug. Or they might just say, in a relieved tone of voice, "Oh, good, Dr. Pezzi is here." Either way, it made me feel welcome and appreciated. It was a great feeling.

▪ I was taking the history on an elderly man when a 3-year-old boy stepped into the cubicle. I'd seen his Mom earlier, and we were awaiting the results of her urinalysis. A cute, precocious youngster with a devilishly appealing charm, he smiled while impatiently tapping his right foot on the ground and said, "Hey, Doc, what's taking so long?" Hmm, good question, I thought. It *had* been quite a while, so I decided to check on the result, and have a little fun at the same time. Stepping out of the cubicle, I told him what to say to the nurse.

With all the confidence and adroitness of a polished Hollywood star, he boldly strode toward the nurse. Crossing his arms over his chest, he leaned back slightly and looked straight into her eyes, saying, "Nurse, we need the results of the urinalysis, *stat!*" Awaiting her reply, which was undoubtedly delayed by a good deal of surprise, he once more resumed tapping his foot, accompanied by a mischievous grin. The nurse slowly looked over at me with an incredulous look on her face, and we all burst out laughing.

▪ "Dr. Pezzi, we have a patient here with hives." Glancing at the patient that the nurse was calling my attention to, I immediately recognized that it was more than hives. Amy's face was swollen, and I determined that her ability to breathe was in serious jeopardy. I helped Amy onto a stretcher, and I ordered the usual medical treatment for this condition. Still, I worried that it may be too late for this, and that I might have to either intubate her (place a tube into her windpipe) or even establish a surgical airway. The latter procedure is what lay people often refer to as a *tracheostomy*; in reality, this procedure is rarely done. Instead, we do an operation termed a *cricothyrotomy*, in which we make an opening just below the voice box, through which a tube is inserted that bypasses the swollen, obstructed airway above.

Amy, who was about 20, was a waitress at a restaurant in a town about ten miles south of the city in which the ER was located. Coincidentally, I lived in the same town, and I'd been to that restaurant, which was known for its good food. On a break, Amy ate some fish to which she was highly allergic.

While I stood by Amy, I had the nurse prepare the equipment I'd need if the medicine didn't act soon. After several anxious minutes, it was clear that she was responding to the treatment, and there was no need for more aggressive intervention. I then admitted her to the hospital for observation, since the effects of the medicine sometimes wear off, resulting in a recrudescence of the original problem.

After she was admitted, I went to visit her to see how she was doing. When I walked into her room, I wondered if I was in the correct room. The patient was slim, and the last time I'd seen Amy, she looked quite bloated. Sure enough, it was her, obviously much better. I spent some time chatting with Amy and her fiancé, then I went back to the ER.

A few years later, I was with my Mom at a restaurant. When the time came to pay the bill, the waitress would not accept my credit card. I began wondering what snafu my credit card company had created, then the waitress said, "Your bill has been taken care of." I was bewildered by this, since I hadn't yet paid the bill, but she once again assured me, "Don't worry, it's already been paid." I looked across the room, and there was Amy, smiling.

▪ After riding my Sea-doo® ("Jet-ski") for a while, I decided to take a break. I sat on the beach while slowly sipping a soft drink, basking in the luxuriant radiation of the sun. A slight breeze caressed my skin, dissipating the small beads of sweat triggered by the August heat. Off in the distance I could hear children playing. In such a perfect world, it was hard to believe that there was a need for emergency rooms. Ah, but they existed, and I'd left one just hours before. But now it was my time to relax, and the day was off to a great start. After stretching out on the warm, sun-bleached sand, I slowly succumbed to the heat. As daydreams melted into dreams, I began to doze off.

I'd occasionally begin to awaken when a boat roared past the beach, but sleep would greet me within seconds. This, however, was different. I sensed that someone was near, but I wasn't conscious enough to care. I thought they would go away, just like the boats, allowing me to resume my nap.

It happened all of a sudden. Feeling soft hands cupped over my eyes, I heard someone say, "Guess who?"

I was startled by this unexpected turn of events, and a fleeting moment of reflexive panic swept over me. But wait, I thought, how many criminals introduce themselves by saying "Guess who?" Precious few, I'm sure. Thus reassured, I turned to face my mystery guest.

Blinking my eyes a few times, she came into focus. Still, I didn't recognize her. My bewilderment must have been apparent. Her voice sounding noticeably less playful, she inquired, "Don't you remember me?"

I wish I had. Her auburn hair framed a face which sent a wave of rapture surging through my spine. Delightful curves accentuated her well-toned body, and her mellifluous voice was friendly and inviting. Then it hit me—I knew her, but not her name. She'd brought her niece to the ER a few weeks ago with a broken clavicle (collar bone). At the time, we had chatted amicably, but I'd never asked for her name. Now I wish I had. "Uh, you're Monica's aunt . . ." Charitably, she completed my sentence. "It's Megan, but you can call me Meg. My friends call me both."

She thanked me for being so nice to Monica. I'd given her a "Get Well" card that I'd made on my computer, and some scratch 'n' sniff stickers I bought from a store in Chicago. She said that Monica kept talking about "that doctor with the Alf puppet." I thought that Monica was too old to be amused by my Alf (remember that old TV show?) animations, but I'd used the puppet to entertain a younger patient in an adjacent bed. Actually, I'd also used the Alf puppet as a diagnostic tool, but that's another story.

A few hours passed. In that time, we were well past the banalities of getting to know one another. It was as if we had known one another for years. In a way, we had. Our dreams and thoughts bore a remarkable similarity, obviating the need for elaborate explanations. No Mars/Venus dichotomy here, I realized.

As the sun dipped in the afternoon sky, Megan suggested riding the Sea-doo®. Like everything else thus far, it was the right thing to do. Since she wanted to drive, I explained the craft's operation. When she ignited the engine, she turned her head around. Smiling, she said, "Well, aren't you going to hold on?" The Sea-doo® had a strap on the seat for the passenger to grip, but I liked her idea better. Her hands grasped mine, which she then wrapped around her waist. Our escalating intimacy was truncated when she hammered the throttle, rocketing the Sea-doo® across the waves. Blown by the wind, wisps of her hair tickled my face. I pulled her closer. She rested her feet on mine, and we danced across the water as she sent the Sea-doo® on graceful spirals. Life couldn't get any better than this, could it?

It could. Entering a deserted bay, she let off the throttle, and stopped the engine. She turned around to face me, undoing the buckles on my life vest which had become nothing but an unwelcome buffer between us. Reflexively, I slipped off her vest, and our lips met as we passionately embraced. Mesmerized by her kissing, we headed for the vacant beach.

As if we both sensed the need to interject some more familiarity before our passion was given free rein, our conversation continued. As the chill of the approaching night slipped upon us, we built a campfire and snuggled before it. "Where do we go from here?" I wondered aloud. Marriage? Children? No. That was not to be. "Cleveland," she responded. "Cleveland?" I asked, more than puzzled. "Yes," she replied matter-of-factly, "my husband was just transferred there."

My spirit instantly wilted, like a dandelion exposed to a nuclear blast. "You're *married*? Where's your wedding ring?"

"I took it off when I saw you." No other explanation was forthcoming.

"Why did you do that?" I inquired.

She began to explain. She said that she was quite taken by my interactions with the pediatric patients that night in the ER. In addition to my Alf routine, she'd heard me singing to another child. This I'd sometimes do to let the child know that the big, scary guy in the white coat was not so scary after all. I'd have never guessed that my crooning would lead to this.

Her husband was intelligent and successful, but crude and unromantic. He was gravy, but she craved honey. She wanted more. She wanted me, she said.

For a man who believed in the sanctity of marriage, her words offered confusion, not clarification. She attempted to explain that this was workable, in spite of how it might seem otherwise. I wasn't buying it. As her words droned on, my ears became increasingly numb. As her image dissolved into an apparition, I got up to leave.

Thanks for the memories, Megan.

# What former patients[32] have said about Dr. Pezzi:

"I want to thank you for helping us, Dr. Pezzi. I have never seen a doctor so interested and dedicated in a long, long time." (Signed, A.H.)

"Dr. Pezzi is a doll; he's so nice." (Telephone survey of an ER patient, G.S.) A letter that she subsequently sent stated, "You are such a sweet and kind, considerate man. I thank you again for being there (Thank God) and being so nice."

(Telephone call from Mrs. A., received by administration.) "Dr. Pezzi was the physician on duty, and Mrs. A. indicated that he was extremely caring and considerate in the treatment of Michele. Mrs. A. was impressed with Dr. Pezzi's efficiency in treating so many people at one time and his low-keyed manner in such a hectic atmosphere."

(Telephone call from Mrs. W., received by administration.) "She called to say how wonderful a doctor Dr. Pezzi was. That she hadn't felt good in months and thanks to Dr. Pezzi she feels much better and will never go to another hospital again. She also stated that if Dr. Pezzi ever moved, she wanted him to send her a card and say where he is going. She said she'll go wherever he goes because he is now her doctor for life."

(Note from M.B., R.N.) "Recently I was in the local grocery store when a woman there noticed my badge. She asked if I worked there and I told her yes. She proceeded to tell me that her husband was a cardiac patient here recently and that he had the most wonderful doctor, his name Dr. Pezzi. She went on to explain how he took the time to explain everything to her and her husband. She also said that he was one of the most caring and thoughtful doctors that she had ever met. She told me we should feel very lucky to have such a wonderful doctor on staff here."

(Telephone call received by administration.) "Michael M. would like to compliment Dr. Pezzi. He thought he was an excellent doctor all the way around—everything from suture repair to pleasant personality. Stated it was the best suture job he ever had."

(Letter from T.F.) "You are an extraordinary man and Doctor, and we feel fortunate to have met you. Remind your patients how lucky they are to have you as their Doc, because _THEY ARE_." (emphasis not added)

(Letter from R.B.) "I was seen in your ER . . . The attending physician was a Dr. Pezzi. He listened to what my symptoms were and looked at some x-rays that I had brought with me from an IVP that I had done the day before at Michigan

---

[32]    *Well, the ones that liked me, anyway!*

Diagnostic. After looking at the x-rays he said that I had a kidney stone in my lower left ureter and it had probably dropped into my bladder. I thought this was amazing because the Dr. at Michigan Diagnostic, a Dr. G., and my own urologist Dr. S. had both missed this stone even though I also told them that whenever I had pains they were always on the lower left side and groin area. Dr. G. even wrote in his report and I quote, "Left kidney and ureter are normal." But Dr. Pezzi was able to find this. In closing I would like to once again thank Dr. Pezzi for being so careful in reading those x-rays and to say what an asset he is for [this] hospital."

"On September 21st, my son's 8th birthday, I brought him to ER to have his lower eyelid sewn up. I wanted to thank you all, especially Dr. Pezzi, for your patience and the great job done on his eye. I have been in the ER quite a few times at various hospitals but this was the first time I was impressed with the staff's performance. Thank you so much for being so understanding when my son was not cooperative at all. Thank you Dr. Pezzi for the wonderful job you did. Larry's eyelid has healed very nicely and it looks good." (Signed, D.M.)

"I would like to express my thanks to you for what I guess you could say your bedside manners. You made me feel very comfortable and were very helpful. Along with this you seemed to make my daughter feel at ease with being in a frightening place to her. I would hope that if I have to return (in a way I would like to[33]), that you would be the doctor that I would get. Again, thank you for the caring that you gave." (Signed, P.W.)

"Thank you again for the care you gave [my daughter] Catherine. I know you are probably told this all the time, but you are one wonderful person and we are very appreciative." (Signed, K.&C.B.)

"My experience with emergency rooms has been, at times, somewhat disappointing when waiting a period of time to see an overworked ER physician who is lacking in either time or interest or both. I cannot express how relieved (and surprised) I was by my visit. I was most especially impressed with the attending physician, Dr. Kevin Pezzi. I have never before experienced such an unhurried manner in an ER physician, and the accompanying feeling for me, as a patient, that he was genuinely interested and concerned in my problem. Furthermore, he was able to immediately diagnose and successfully treat a condition for which my own physician had not done the same. I have on very few occasions felt the trust and confidence in *any* physician after so little time that Dr. Pezzi immediately instilled. Though my experience with Dr. Pezzi was limited and very brief, I would recommend him most favorably at any opportunity. My only regret is that he is, as an ER physician, not available in private practice, because he would most certainly be my regular physician if he were. I hope that you appreciate Dr. Pezzi . . ." (Signed, A.L.)

---

[33]    *Imagine actually **wanting** to return to an Emergency Room!*

# Comments about Dr. Pezzi's
## *Fascinating Health Secrets*

**Registered Nurse, Flint, MI:** "Wow! What a book! How much does it cost? No, I don't care how much—I've got to have that book!"

**Eye Doctor, Phoenix, AZ:** "It's fantastic—I couldn't put the book down!"

**David Hacker,** *Prime Time News & Observer*: "There's an odd fascination with the way Pezzi's mind works. He is a scholar, bright (possibly brilliant), and single-minded. There's plenty of useful information . . . some interesting tidbits . . . life-saving tips . . . and amusing historic trivia. For the most part, you can take this book seriously. At the same time, you can have fun with its folksy, whimsical and chatty style."

**Alan Jakeway,** *Northern Express*: "You've got to hand it to Dr. Pezzi—he knows how to craft a health book that's as gripping as a ride through a big city ER. While many health books are as dry and dull as a surgeon's medical transcript, Dr. Pezzi brings a good bedside manner to his book, blending humor, first-person insights and a folksy wisdom with cutting edge medicine. *Fascinating Health Secrets* is a "good read" page-turner that will keep your attention at the beach as well as any summer novel."

**Bookstore Owner, Gaylord, MI:** "I loved the book. Before I read it, I thought it was going to be dry—but it wasn't."

**Reader, Las Vegas, NV:** ". . . a refreshing change from the insipid writing in other health books. Keep up the good work."

**Stockbroker, Mobile, AL:** "It's got a lot of appeal, that book."

**Paralegal, Lapeer, MI:** "This is really cool! A neat book!"

**Accountant, Grand Blanc, MI:** "My entire family has read your book, and they all want a copy for themselves—it's unique."

**ABC News Reporter:** "Fantastic book!"

**Emergency Dispatcher, Greenbelt, MD:** "I picked up the book at the post office, and I started reading it in the car in the parking lot. Pretty soon, about 15 minutes flew by! I decided to get back home before I stayed there all day. Your ER stories put Michael Crichton (creator of the TV show "ER") to shame. You recount your stories quite vividly."

**Retired Dentist, Albion, MI:** "That book by Dr. Pezzi is fabulous. You would expect a man who is such an unusually bright person would be beyond the average person to understand. He is so down-to-earth and practical, so sensible and honest. I wish he was practicing here—I would go to him in a minute. That's one book that won't be loaned to anyone."

**Magazine Editor/Columnist, Dunlap, IL:** "I find it really enjoyable, an easy read with lots of interesting facts, opinions and fun stuff."

**Airline Industry Analyst, Ft. Worth, TX:** "Most authors content themselves giving you the same old platitudes, apparently thinking that it's better to bore you than to risk offending a small segment of the population. What I found most refreshing is that Dr. Pezzi has the guts to say what needs to be said."

**Reader, Roscommon, MI:** "I am so glad you aspired to become a doctor. I am even more thrilled that you decided to share some of your wisdom via a book. *Fascinating Health Secrets* is incredibly interesting with many real-life applications. Your book is an outstanding resource. I am already looking forward to the next book. You did an excellent job of pinning down and sorting out a wealth of information."

**Reader, Age 68, Houghton Lake, MI:** "This is the first book in my life that I've read cover-to-cover."

**Will Brink, Health & Fitness Author and Magazine Columnist:** "This is a really cool book full of all sorts of interesting information . . . full of facts and humor."

**And from a reader in Bellevue, WA:** "*Loved* your book!"

---

**You wouldn't think that a person who has access to some of the best doctors in the world would have a need for this book, right?**

**Trivia question: Which celebrity owns two copies of *Fascinating Health Secrets*?**

Answer: Vice-president Al Gore.

# *Fascinating Health Secrets*

Intriguing tips on medicine, beauty, health,
sleep, nutrition, weight loss, longevity, exercise,
brainpower, sexual attraction, and sex

ISBN 0-9655606-0-0
476 pages, including index
*a TRANSCOPE Publication*

---

*Fascinating Health Secrets* **includes a number of
emergency room stories which are not present in**
*Believe It or Not! TRUE Emergency Room Stories*, **in
addition to thousands of health tips—many of which
you won't find in other books!**

---

*To order, send a check or money order to:*
Transcope, Inc.
955 Nature Trail
Holly, MI 48442

*If you would like your book autographed by the author, please mention this with your order.*

## *Price*

U.S.: $19.95 (plus $3 Priority Mail shipping) = $22.95 total
*Michigan residents must add $1.20 sales tax ($24.15 total)*

Canada: $27.50 (plus $1.85 book rate shipping) = $29.35 total *or*
Canada: $27.50 (plus $6.95 Global Priority Mail shipping) = $34.45 total

*Priority Mail shipping (to the U.S. or Canada) is free if
you order more than one item (see the next page).*

---

Dr. Pezzi will answer questions from readers by personal mail.
Enclose a check (made out to *Transcope, Inc.*) for $30.00 per question.
Dr. Pezzi is also available for seminars; write to the address given
above.

## Believe It or Not! TRUE Emergency Room Stories

is also available excerpted on audio tapes (two 90-minute
cassettes; approximately 3 hours running time).

---

To order the audio cassettes or another copy of the book (the
price of each is the same), send a check or money order to:

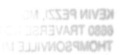

Transcope, Inc.
955 Nature Trail
Holly, MI 48442

*Be sure to specify if you want the audio cassettes or the book.*

*If you are ordering the book and would like it autographed by
the author, please mention this with your order.*

## Price

### 1st Class shipping

U.S.: $12.95 (plus $1.50 First Class Mail) = $14.45 total

*Michigan residents must add 78 cents sales tax ($15.23 total)*

### Priority Mail shipping

U.S.: $12.95 (plus $3 Priority Mail shipping) = $15.95 total

*Michigan residents must add 78 cents sales tax ($16.73 total)*

**Canada:** $17.50 (plus $1.37 book rate shipping) = $18.87 total *or*
**Canada:** $17.50 (plus $6.95 Global Priority Mail shipping) = $24.45 total

**Priority Mail shipping (to the U.S. _or_ Canada) is free if
you order more than one item (see the preceding page).**

---

Dr. Pezzi will answer questions from readers by personal mail.
Enclose a check (made out to *Transcope, Inc.*) for $30.00 per question.
Dr. Pezzi is also available for seminars; write to the address given
above.

If the reader response card is missing, please fill out this form and mail it to Transcope, Inc., 955 Nature Trail, Holly, MI 48442. *Thank you!*

> *Register your purchase, and we will send you a coupon good for 10% off your next order.*

**Product(s) purchased:**
☐ *Fascinating Health Secrets*
☐ *Believe It or Not! TRUE Emergency Room Stories* (audio cassettes)
☐ *Believe It or Not! TRUE Emergency Room Stories* (CD)
☐ *Believe It or Not! TRUE Emergency Room Stories* (book)
**Place of purchase:**

---

| Name of store or catalogue | City | State |

**Your comments are greatly appreciated:**
(continue on reverse side if you need additional space)

*May we quote you in promotional material?* YES   NO   (please circle)

Your name and address

If you would like to be notified by e-mail when Dr. Pezzi has published new books, please include your e-mail address.

A mailing label for your convenience: ➡

**TRANSCOPE, INC.**
**955 NATURE TRAIL**
**HOLLY, MI 48442**

KEVIN PEZZI, MD
6680 TRAVERSE ROAD
THOMPSONVILLE MI 49683